STABILITY BALL EXERCISES

Fitness and Performance Exercises

For Strength, Stability and Flexibility

STABILITY BALL EXERCISES

Fitness and Performance Exercises for

Strength, Stability and Flexibility

Marina Aagaard, MFE

Aarhus, Denmark

aagaard | marina aagaard

STABILITY BALL EXERCISES

Fitness and Performance Exercises for Strength, Stability and Flexibility

1. edition, 1. impression

ISBN 978-87-92693-53-2

Editor: Marina Aagaard

Graphic design: Marina Aagaard

Photography: Marina Aagaard, Henrik Elstrup

Cover photography: Claus Petersen, CPhotography, www.cphotography.com

Printer: Lulu.com

aagaard | marina aagaard

www.marinaaaagaard.dk

Contents

Preface

Welcome to *Stability ball Exercises*. A comprehensive reference book for stability ball exercises for individual, partner and group exercise.

The book is intended for coaches, trainers, instructors, physiotherapists as well as physical education teachers and students with some basic knowledge of physiology and training. Many good books cover the prerequisites for exercise selection and programme design. This book is dedicated to giving you with as many stability ball exercises as possible.

The book presents stability ball exercises at all levels, from very easy exercises used in rehabilitation and recreational exercise to advanced exercises used by Olympic athletes. This gives coaches, trainers and instructors more options and assists in progressing exercise programmes in better and more motivating ways.

Often trainers and therapists habitually use the same exercises over and over again, but there is a demand for new and varied exercises in order to provide mental and physical variation and stimulation to the people you coach, train and teach.

An important purpose of this book is to make it easier and more expedient to find the specific exercise you are looking for. It accomplishes this by bringing together a multitude of exercises at all levels from different training millieus: Exercises with just your bodyweight and the ball, exercises with different pieces of equipment and ball exercises with a partner.

The prime goal is to provide stability ball exercises for workouts, which are safe, specific, time-efficient and enjoyable for all involved.

I wish you good reading and good training.

Marina Aagaard, 2011

Aknowledgements

I am grateful for the many people who helped in making this book possible: My husband, family and friends for supporting and encouraging me.

Thanks to all of you who provided inspiration, ideas and feedback throughout the years, colleagues and students at the Academy of Coaching, Aalborg Sportshoejskole, colleagues and students at Aalborg University, professors and fellow students at The University of Southern Denmark, fellow intercontinental FIG coaches and friends at the Danish Gymnastics Federation.

Special thanks to the fitness models, the energetic and patient trainers who helped in making this book come to life:

Physiotherapist Heidi Tang Moeller
Diploma fitness coach Astrid Kirkegaard and Kirstine Kirkegaard, stud. med.
Diploma strength training coach Morten Kirstein

Marina Aagaard, 2011

1 | How to Use This Book

Stability Ball Exercises is an important resource for coaches, trainers, instructors, physiotherapists and PE teachers using the stability ball, also known *as the Swiss ball, core ball, physio ball, strength ball, resistance ball* or *therapy ball.* With exercises for sports, gymnastics, general fitness, one-on-one or small group training, and group exercise.

Some basic knowledge of anatomy, physiology and exercise science is needed to select, sequence and execute the exercises correctly. Do not progress without the help of a fitness professional, if you are unfamiliar with stability ball training.
Important: All exercises are meant for average healthy exercisers free from any serious or disabilitating disease, illness or ailments. Please consult your doctor before beginning these exercises.

Programme design – number of sets and repetitions, duration of rest-pauses and speed of movement – is not discussed, as many other books cover these areas in detail.
Program design will vary with the goal of the exercise and the skill and strength level of the exerciser. However, for general fitness 1-3 sets of 6-12 repetitions of 6-10 ball exercises are appropriate. The exercise tempo should be moderate and rest-pauses around ½-2 minutes.

The exercises are listed by muscle groups and in most instances after increasing level of difficulty. However, there are some exceptions, as many factors play a role.
The book contains exercises at all levels from introductory to advanced – for novices with no previous exercise experience, beginners with no ball training experience, and intermediate to advanced exercisers, who are skilled and strong.

The first chapters cover basic information and warm-up exercises. The following chapters cover stability ball exercises for the upper body, the lower body and the core. The last chapters cover ball exercises with additional equipment, ball exercises with a partner and stretches with the stability ball. All the information you need to create a complete and balanced ball workout.

2 | Stability Ball Basics

The stability ball is one of the most versatile pieces of equipment within exercise and fitness. It provides an endless array of fun and effective exercises for all target groups, juniors, adults and seniors.

The stability ball is an indispensable piece of equipment for balance and core work. Both areas are fundamental in improving the quality of life – and performance in sports.
This along with a number of other advantages means, that stability ball training is a fixture in so-called functional training as an excellent exercise modality complimentary to working out on a stable surface.

Ball types

There a two primary **types of balls, regular and ABS**, *Anti Burst System*. Regular balls can be used for most exercises, and are especially suited for exercises with bouncing and hopping movements on on the stability ball. However, they are better for lighter loads and may burst instantaneously, if they come in contact with something sharp and then puncture.

If you take good care of your regular ball, some of which have been tested up to several hundred kilos, and you follow the guidelines for pumping and handling the ball, they are quite durable, so do not worry; they will not burst too easily.

For training with larger loads, for exercises standing on the ball and for exercises with free weights, ABS stability balls are recommended: ABS balls do not burst, when punctured, but deflate gradually. Also they are quite thick; some are tested up to loads of 500 kilos.
They are not quite as lively as the regular balls, so they are easier to balance (and stand) on.

The ballsize

For exercising **the recommended ballsize depends on height, bodyweight, body position and the type of exercise**. Also the length of the limbs is a factor; if your arms or legs are very short or very long, this will affect, which ballsize is better.

Even if there are some common guidelines for choosing the right ballsize, both juniors and adults – independently of height – may use both smaller and larger balls than recommended for certain exercises and games, e.g. very large balls of 150 and 180 centimeter Ø, MegaBalls from Gymnic™.

Smaller balls are suited for exercises, where 1) the stability ball are held between the legs, eg. hip adduction, or under the legs, hamstring curl, and for 2) push-up's, where the legs support on the stability ball, 3) sidelying exercises and 4) plank exercises with the feet on the stability ball.

Larger balls are suited for 1) use as a chair, 2) seated exercises, 3) stretching, 4) weight training exercises, to avoid that the weight touches the floor during upperbody exercises, and 5) exercises, where you roll across the stability ball.

If you have a ball, that is too big for your body or exercise, you can let out some of the air. You may still use the ball, even if it is a bit softer.

If you have a ball, that is too small, you cannot inflate it to more than the recommended ball size, as the ball will burst! Instead get another ball or do some other exercises.

Finding the right ball size:

Sit on the ball with the feet flat on the ground. The hips and knees should at least be at a 90 degreess angle, so the thighs are parallel to the floor, or better, a little above.

If the stability ball is too small, with the thighs below horizontal during seated exercises, this may lead to a poor posture, slouching on the ball.

Recommended size of stability ball, diameter Ø	
45 cm	< 155 cm
55 cm	150-172 cm
65 cm	165-188 cm
75 cm	180-198 cm
85 cm	> 198 cm

Inflating the ball

When getting a new stability ball, first of all read the instructions to ensure proper inflation and handling of the ball. This is important to prevent that the stability ball bursts. **Maximal ballsize, which is printed on the stability ball, must not be exceeded.**

The stability ball can be inflated with a suitable 2-way hand- or footpump or an air compressor. It is almost impossible to inflate the stability ball with the mouth. Using a bicycle pump is also a slow and difficult means of inflating the ball.

The compressor pumps the ball very quickly and is recommended, if you have a lot of balls to inflate, but be very careful not to over inflate the ball. Note: Air compressors blow cold air that could expand after returning to room temperature!

To ensure that the stability ball is not over inflated check the diameter with a (folding) ruler. Do this by measuring and marking the ball diameter on a wall and hold the ruler perpendicular to this. This makes it easy to see, when the ball has the right size.

The stability ball diameter should match the recommended size printed on the ball and be firm, but not too firm. When you put a finger to the ball, the ball surface should deform slightly corresponding to a hollowing of approx. 2 inches (4-5 cm) in diameter.

Before inflating the ball, make sure the ball has room temperature and then

1) inflate it to 80 % of its size (your finger can make a hollowing of 6 inches (15 cm) Ø),

2) let it rest for a couple hours or more – I recommend 24 hours – and then

3) inflate it completely, and

4) let the stability ball rest for 24 hours before using it.

'Softer', not fully inflated balls do not roll around as much, which makes the exercises easier to perform. A softer ball is recommended for novices, the elderly and weaker target groups. Firm fully inflated balls are more lively, suited for intermediate to advanced exercisers.

The ball should be inflated approximately every third to fourth month depending on how often it is used. It is easy: Hand- and footpumps are cheap and can inflate the stability ball in 1-2 minutes. Take out the valve with a teaspoon, no sharp instrument (!), when you wish to inflate or deflate the ball.

Handling, Storing and Cleaning

Take good care of your stability ball:

- Keep the stability ball free of dust, pebbles, debris and sharp objects.

- The floor must be clean, no sand, pebbles or glass, that will scratch or puncture the ball.

- Avoid scratching the ball with jewellery or watches. Do not wear these, when ball training.

- Wear only clean indoor shoes or bare feet, when ball training.

- Do not kick or throw the stability ball as it may puncture. Handle with care.

- The stability ball is only for indoor use, if you want it to last. If you want to use it outdoors, use a mat underneath the ball.

- Store at room temperature, not strong heat and cold, which will affect the ball (do not store in a car, outdoor shed or the attic). Avoid exposure to extreme variations in temperature. Avoid direct sunlight, do not place in front of windows or other heat sources.

- Hold the ball up against the light to see, if there are anywhere, where the light shines through, weaker parts of the ball, which may result in the ball puncturing during training.

- Clean the stability ball with a soft cloth. Use only warm water or a mild detergent. Do not use any kind of solvents, abrasive or chemical cleaners.

- A punctured ball cannot hold air, so it must be thrown out. There is no use in trying to mend it, because it will not last.

- The stability balls will keep for many years with proper care. However, with heavy duty use, some experts recommend changing the ball every year or every other year.

3 | Technique and Safety

In order to maximize your workout benefit and minimize ineffecient use of your time or even risk of injuries, this chapter sums up the main points of good exercise technique.

The exercise tables only list general and special points for exercise technique. In all exercises a **good posture is a prerequisite**: A strong and stable body with timely controlled contraction of the core muscles, a.o. pelvic floor and transversus abdominis.

Depending on the exercise, this should be limited to either one primary muscle, as in isolation exercises, or a number of muscles, compound exercises, in one controlled movement. In any exercise you should *avoid unwanted co-movements, such as the head and shoulder girdle dropping forward, excessive arching or hunching of the lower back, and locking of the knees or elbows.*

Breathing should be deep 'abdominal' breathing. Inhale through the nose and exhale through the nose or mouth.

The typical resistance training breathing pattern is biomechanical breathing: Inhale on the eccentric phase of the exercise and exhale on the concentric phase for greater force production.

Anatomical breathing: You inhale when you extend the back, opening up your ribcage allowing for more air into the lungs, and exhale when you bend, reducing space for air.

During all exercises keep breathing; this will increase the energy and enhance the workout.

The ball exercises should be preceded by a warm-up of 5-20 minutes depending on the intensity and duration of the workout.

Programme design will vary with the goal of the exercise and the skill and strength level of the exerciser. However, stability ball training for general fitness normally comprises 1-3 sets of 6-12 repetitions of 6-10 ball exercises. Exercise tempo should be slow to moderate initially and rest-pauses last ½-2 minutes. Exercise should be followed by a cooldown, of 3-5 minutes depending of the intensity and the exerciser. Include relevant stretches as needed.

Basic posture

Initiate all workouts and exercises with a good posture: The prerequisite for optimal results.

Front view: Image a plumb line through the middle of the body. Head and neck, shoulders and hips should form a symmetrical image around this line.

Side view: Image a plumb line passing through the ear, shoulder, hip, knee and ankle (just in front of the outer malleol bone).

If you see significant deviations from this, you need to correct the posture or do some exercises, that will help you obtain a better posture. In some instances you need to have a physiotherapist perform relevant testing and provide the necessary corrective exercises.

Standing starting position

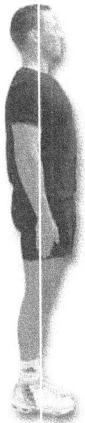

Focus points:

- Legs together or hip- or shoulder-width apart.
- Feet forward or a little outward.
- Feet are firmly positioned with the weight evenly distributed across the foot; keep the heel and toes on the ground.
- Knees are aligned with feet; knee aligned with the second toe.
- Knees are relaxed, not locked, hyperextended, or overly flexed.
- Pelvis is in a neutral position.
- Transversus abdominis contraction as needed to stabilize.
- The spine is in neutral position with a natural curve.
- Shoulder blades are in neutral.
- Shoulders are lowered and level.
- Neck is in neutral position.
- Tongue rests in the roof of the mouth behind the front teeth.

Seated starting position

Focus points:

- Legs are either wide apart, shoulder- or hip-width apart or together (depending on skill level, the exercise and how much you want to challenge your balance).
- Feet are firmly positioned on the floor.
- Knees are aligned with feet.
- Contract the pelvic floor muscles.
- Contract the transversus abdominis to stabilize the body as needed.
- Hips are level, also during one leg supports.
- Spine is in neutral position.
- Shoulder blades are in neutral position.
- Shoulders are level and lowered.
- Neck is in neutral position.
- Tongue rests in the roof of the mouth behind the front teeth
- Hands are on the ball, the legs or at the waist.

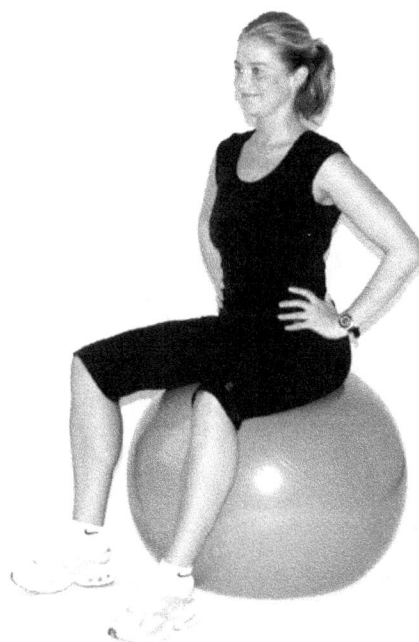

Supine starting position

Focus points:

- Legs are either wide apart, shoulder- or hip-width apart or together
  (depending on skill level, the exercise and how much you want to challenge your balance).
- Feet are firmly positioned on the floor.
- Knees are aligned with the feet.
- Contract the pelvic floor muscles.
- Contract the transversus abdominis to stabilize the body.
- Hips are level, also during one leg supports.
- Spine is in neutral position, with a natural curve of the spine.
- The lower back rests across the top of the stability ball, so the navel is right above the top
  of the ball. This is the starting position for traditionel ab curls at intermediate level.
  Point of support: The shoulder blades. Do not rest on the neck.
- Shoulder blades are in neutral position, not forwards or outwards.
- Shoulders are level and lowered.
- Neck is in neutral position.
- Tongue rests in the roof of the mouth behind the front teeth
- Hands are on the thighs, by the side of the body, at the chest or the side of the head.

- *Note: Some exercisers find it uncomfortable to have the torso and head too far back.*
  Exercisers may experience, that they lose their bearing, feel heated or a little dizzy.
  Therefore a good starting position is an incline, semi-recumbent position (left photo),
  where the torso is more upright. From here you can gradually move further back.
  Note: Hold and stabilize the ball with the hands in order to avoid, that it rolls backwards.

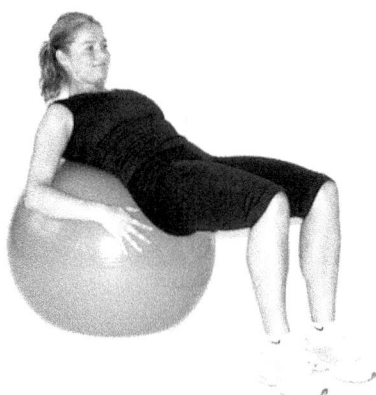

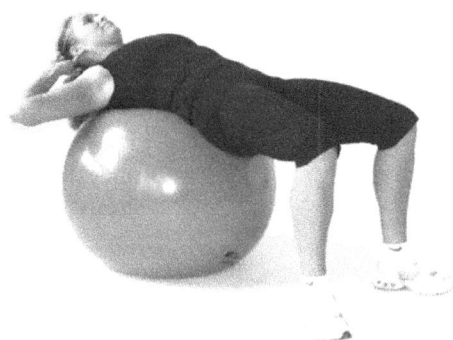

Prone starting position

Focus points:

- Legs are either wide apart, shoulder- or hip-width apart or together
  (depending on skill level, the exercise and how much you want to challenge your balance).
- Toes are firmly on the floor.
- Knees are aligned with the feet.
- Contract the pelvic floor muscles.
- Contract the transversus abdominis to stabilize the body.
- Hips are level, also during one leg supports.
  The abdomen rests across the top of the ball, so the navel is right above the top.
  Depending on height, leg length and ballsize you may have to shift the position for better balance on the ball.
- Shoulder blades are in neutral position.
- Shoulders are level and lowered.
- Neck is in neutral position.
- Tongue rests in the roof of the mouth behind the front teeth
- Hands are on the floor, on the ball, on the chest or by the side of the head.

- Get up slowly, when going from prone to standing position to avoid getting dizzy.

- *Note: When the hands are on the floor, eg. during plank positions or walk-outs, it may be uncomfortable for the wrists. This is because the wrists are small joints and it is not common to support your bodyweight on them during everyday living. Therefore the wrists must be strengthened gradually during the exercises. Until they are stronger, use slow, controlled movements and avoid doing too many repetitions, holding isometric exercises for too long or putting too much weight on them (eg. lever arm too long).*

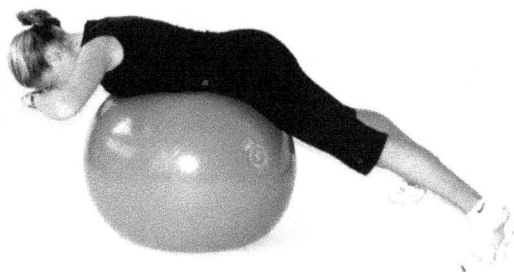

Sidelying starting position

Focus points:

- Legs are straight. Or the lower leg is bent and on the floor (easier; left photo).
- Legs are staggered, wide apart or right in front of each other. Or above one another. *Note: In the sidelying position it may be better to have the feet on an exercise mat or a yoga mat to prevent the feet from slipping.*
- Knees are aligned with the feet.
- Contract the pelvic floor muscles.
- Contract the transversus abdominis to stabilize the body.
- Hips are in line, avoid rolling forwards or backwards.
- The waist is on top of the stability ball, so the navel is centered approx. above the top of the ball. This is the starting position for traditional sidebending obliques exercises.
- Shoulder blades are in neutral position.
- Neck is in neutral position. *Note: In the sidelying position you have a tendency to lift the head sidewards to vertical position. Keep the head in line with the spine.*
- Tongue rests in the roof of the mouth behind the front teeth
- Bottom hand on the floor or on the ball. Top arm rests along the side of the body.
- Get up slowly, when going from prone to standing position to avoid getting dizzy.

- *Note: When supporting on one hand, it may be hard on the wrist, especially if you lose balance and there is too much weight on the hand. More so because the wrists are small joints and it is not common to support your bodyweight on them during everyday living. Therefore the wrists must be strengthened gradually during the exercises. Until they are stronger, use slow, controlled movements and avoid doing too many repetitions, holding isometric exercises too long or putting too much weight on the wrist.*

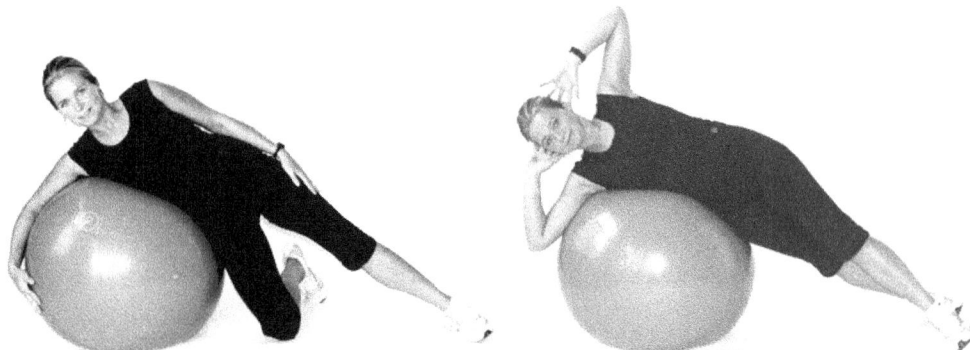

Safety tips

Stability ball training cannot be learned just be reading about it. Be cautious and progress gradually. Have professional instruction the first couple of times.

Focus points for maximum safety, well-being and results during stability ball training:

- Check with your doctor. Stability ball training is recommended for most people, but certain risk factors, diseases or handicaps – or pregnancy – may mean that some exercises have to be modified.

- Weaker participants, the blind, weak-sighted or people with very poor sense of balance, should have a qualified trainer or therapist present to assist.

- Always start with the easiest exercises first to get accustomed to the ball, learn the technique and improve the balance before attempting to perform more difficult exercises. This way you avoid falls and accidents – and loosing courage.

- If during the workout you feel any pain or discomfort, stop immediately. The exercise should then be modified or abandoned, depending on the problem.

- Wrists need to strengthened for stability ball training. Start by doing fewer repetitions with lower load (less weight on the hands) and have frequent rest-pauses.

- Knees may be overloaded or twisted during deep squatting and rotation. Avoid this by contracting the thigh muscles to control the move and keep the knees and feet aligned.

- Do not eat or drink immediately before or during the stability ball workout. It is uncomfortable being on the ball, prone or supine, if the stomach is full.

- The stability ball compresses the abdomen somewhat during prone exercises; it may feel uncomfortable. You get used to being on the ball. Until then contract the abs a little and avoid lying too heavily on the ball. Take frequent breaks to ease the pressure.

- During some supine exercises the back is slightly hyperextended and the abdomen fully stretched; it may feel uncomfortable. It helps to 1) contract the transversus abdominis, 2) avoid lying to long in this position and 3) limit the range of motion.

- Some exercisers may feel nauseous, when the torso is stretched or the head hangs down. This feeling normally disappears. Some exercisers may still feel it occasionally. In these instances limit the range of motion or take a break.

- In case of dizziness, stop and get up slowly to a sitting position and slowly get off the ball. To avoid dizziness limit the range of motion, so the torso and the head do not go too far back or forward.

- Some days the balance is not as good as usual. Then you just stick to an easier exercise to avoid falling. Next time you are ready to move on again.

- When going from one exercise to another, a *transition*, concentrate on this and move in a slow and controlled tempo. Most falls happens during transitions!

- Clear plenty of room around the stability ball. There should be room for the body, the arms and legs to move freely in all directions and if the stability ball is meant to move during the workout, there must be plenty of room for this, too. In exercises with some risk of losing balance, there must be adequate clearence for the ball *and* the exerciser.

- The floor must not be slippery, when ball training. Clean it and/or use a mat or yoga mat as underlay. Be careful when pressing the legs down and the body backwards: If the floor, ball or clothes are slippery, the stability ball may shoot out backwards, so you fall onto the floor. Ensure that the ball is in place and stable on the floor before leaning onto it.

- The clothes for stability ball training should be comfortable. Not too tight or too loose, so it gets in the way. The material should not be too 'slippery', as this can lead to sliding off the stability ball. Avoid long hair being caught by the stability ball.

- Wear only indoor footwear during stability ball training and be careful to wipe of the soles before stepping on the ball surface, so the stability ball does not puncture. Alternatively train in bare feet.

- During standing exercises on the stability ball, use indoor training shoes. If you wear socks or tights you may slip and harm yourself. Bare feet work well with the stability ball, but if you want to stand on the ball, the feet must be dry, not sweaty.

- Wipe off any sweat from the stability ball, so you do not fall off.

Stability ball Progressions

1. Base of support: First arms and hands and/or feet and legs wide apart, then closer together. The wider apart, the easier the exercise, and vice versa.

2. Points of support: First more points of support, then fewer. With both arms and legs, then only one arm and/or leg at a time.

3. With or without support: Feet and/or hands on the floor or ball, then lifted; unsupported.

4. Area of support: First larger, then smaller. Eg. prone on the ball, progression: Support on the thighs, then the lower legs, the feet, the toes.

5. Lever: First body and limbs close to the stability ball, short lever, then longer lever: Eg. plank position with forearms on the ball, progression: Support on the lower legs with the hips flexed, support on the lower legs with the hips straight, support on the toes with legs in straddle position, support on the toes with legs together.

6. Planes. First sagittal plane movements, then diagonal, transversal plane, movements.

7. Vision: First with the eyes open, then one eye closed, then both eyes closed.

8. Centre of gravity. Body position, centre of gravity. First sitting, prone and supine exercises. Then on all fours, kneeling and maybe even standing exercises on the stability ball. *Note: Standing exercises on the stability ball should not be attempted unless you are a skilled exerciser. When getting up onto and when standing on the ball, contract the core muscles at all times and concentrate. Otherwise you may lose balance in a split second and fall off the ball and maybe injure yourself. Be very careful.*

9. Complexity. At first simple, isolated exercises, then compound, complex exercises and then difficult and sports specific exercises on the ball, eg. throws, swings etc.).

10. Stability ball characteristics. Apart from these variations, you can use a softer, not fully inflated ball in the beginning, as this makes the exercises easier. Later on use a harder, fully inflated ball, which is more lively and challenging.

4 | Warm-up and Cardio Moves

In this section there is a selection of warm-up and cardio moves with the stability ball for stability ball training workouts. Build your warm-up around these for variety and intensity.

Warm-up

For stability ball workouts you may choose to warm up by doing easy walking, cycling or low-impact aerobics or using cardio machines like rowers or crosstrainers.

If you use the ball for warming up, keep it simple, as most exercisers into stability ball training want a resistance and balance training workout, not complex choreography.
For group exercise classes you may choose to do a more choreographed warm-up, if the group would enjoy this.

Independantly of the previous warm-up activity it is recommended to do a series of specific torso and pelvic movements immediately before the resistance exercises: Sitting on the ball: Spinal flexion and extension, sideflexion right and left and rotation.
Pelvic tilts, forward and backward, pelvic side tilts and pelvic twists (very small movements in the transversal plane).

Cardio work

Stability ball training will not provide a high-intensity cardio workout. However, it is possible to get the heart rate up and get some cardio work depending on your selection of exercises, the range of motion and the degree of travelling.
For certain target groups, eg. beginners, deconditioned exercisers and the elderly, there may even be a notable cardiovascular effect.

Note: For advanced exercisers certain movements, eg. rolling back and forth across the ball with large total body movements, is an option, that will get the heart rate up.

Warm-up tips

- Instructors: Start with a brief presentation of you, the warm-up and the workout.
- The warm-up should prepare the participant(s) mentally as well as physically.
- It is imperative to make the participant(s) feel at ease with the ball.

- Warm up with or without music.
- Warm up for 5-15 minutes.
- You may extend the warm-up into a longer cardio section or an actual cardio workout.
- Face the particpant(s) to ensure they are happy, comfortable and stable on the ball.
- Tailor the warm-up to the needs and skill level of the participant(s).
- Keep the exercises simple, enjoyable and specific to the content and purpose of the workout.
- Perform a variety of movements to prepare the spine and major joints for the workout; flexion, extension, sideflexion, abduction, adduction and rotation.
- Perform the exercises at a moderate tempo, with occasional tempo or rhythm changes if desired.
- Start with legs wide to provide a good, stable base of support. Then gradually move the legs closer and start lifting the legs one at a time, eg. walking steps and kneelifts.
- Start with a small range of motion and gradually make the movements larger.
- Gradually increase the work load from low to moderate intensity.
- If you do a cardio workout, perform rehearsal moves during the warm-up to learn the names and patterns of the coming moves.

Before starting: The ball exercises in this book are for healthy exercisers. See your doctor before beginning any new exercise modality or get help and instruction from a proficient ball trainer or instructor the first couple of times.

MARCH	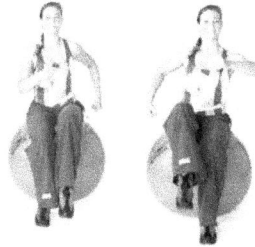
HAMSTRING CURL	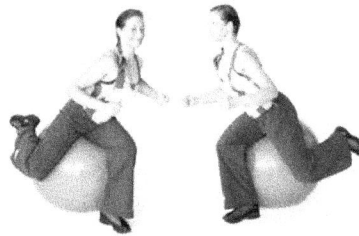
SKIP	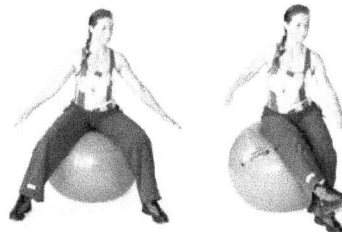
KNEELIFT	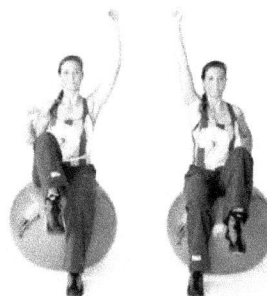

Sit on the ball. Torso erect. Feet on the floor. Walk on the spot. Dynamic arm movements.	Basic warm up and cardio exercise. Can be varied in numerous ways. Bounce on the ball for higher intensity. Contract the core muscles to stabilize.	Without arm movements. With various arm movements. With the eyes closed. Walk forward and backward. Walk side to side, step touch. Walk in a pattern, eg. V-steps. While seated, walk the feet 1/1 circle around the ball.
Sit on the ball. Torso erect. Step a little to the side and bend the knee of the free leg, like a low impact jog. Dynamic arm movements. Repeat with the other leg.	It is a good idea to include some moves for the back of the legs, however this move is somewhat difficult, as the ball is in the way. You must angle your body to be able to curl. Suggestion: Do standing hamstring curls. Contract the core to stabilize.	Without arm movements. With various arm movements. Singles or repeaters.
Sit on the ball. Torso erect. Extend one knee and plantarflex the ankle, point the toes down. Make a small skip. Dynamic arm movements. Repeat with the other leg.	Basic warm up exercise. Can be varied in numerous ways. Bounce on the ball for higher intensity. Contract the thigh to control the movement and protect the knee. Contract the core to stabilize.	Without arm movements. With various arm movements. Skip to the side, forward or in front of the opposite leg. With the eyes closed. Singles or repeaters.
Sit on the ball. Torso erect. Lift one knee up to or above horizontal, hip and knee flexion. Dynamic arm movements. Repeat with the other leg.	Basic warm up exercise. Can be varied in numerous ways. Bounce on the ball for higher intensity. Contract the core muscles to stabilize.	Without arm movements. With various arm movements. Lift the arm overhead and turn the head and look up to the hand – for balance work. With the eyes closed. Singles or repeaters.

KICK

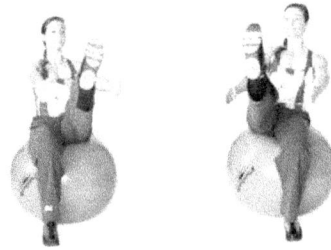

HEELJACK

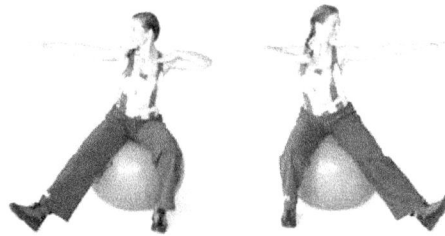

JACK

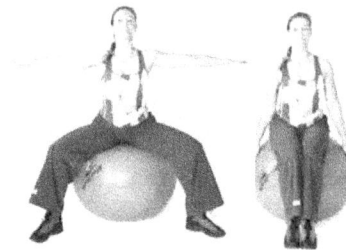

LUNGE

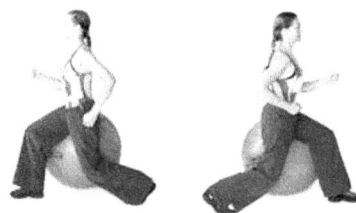

Sit on the ball. Torso erect. Lift one leg up, hip flexion, leg above horizontal, and extend the knee. Or, if possible, keep the leg straight throughout the movement; lifting-lowering. Dynamic arm movements. Repeat with the other leg.	Intermediate warm up exercise. Can be varied in numerous ways. Bounce on the ball for higher intensity. Contract the core muscles to stabilize.	Without arm movements. With various arm movements. With the eyes closed. Singles or repeaters.
Sit on the ball. Torso erect. Lift and abduct the legs, as in a jumping jack, but with one leg bent and foot on the floor and other leg straight and to the side with the heel on the floor. Dynamic arm movements. Adduct and repeat with the other leg straight.	Intermediate warm up exercise. Bounce on the ball for higher intensity. Keep knees and feet aligned, no rotation of the knees. Contract the core, including the pelvic floor, to stabilize.	Without arm movements. With various arm movements. With the eyes closed. Singles or repeaters.
Sit on the ball. Torso erect. Lift and abduct the legs to the side, bent legs and feet on the floor, jumping jack. Adduct the legs, feet together. Dynamic arm movements. Repeat.	Basic warm up exercise. Bounce on the ball for higher intensity. Keep knees and feet aligned, no rotation of the knees. Contract the core, including the pelvic floor muscles, to stabilize.	Without arm movements. With various arm movements. With the eyes closed. Amplitude changes. Rhythm changes and hop combinations.
Sit on the ball. Torso erect. Lift the body and turn to the side, 1/4 hop, and land in lunge position with the feet slightly apart and staggered. Hop or step back to the starting position, 1/4 hop back. Adduct the legs, feet together. Dynamic arm movements. Repeat to the other side.	Advanced warm up exercise. Bounce on the ball for higher intensity. Watch the knees and feet, they should be aligned; avoid rotation of the knees. Contract the core muscles to stabilize.	Without arm movements. With various arm movements. Amplitude changes.

HOP

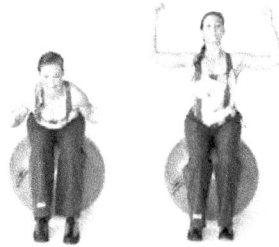

TWIST

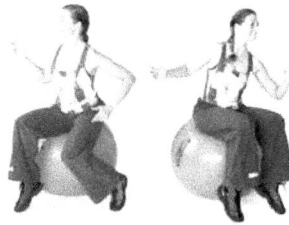

SIDESTEP

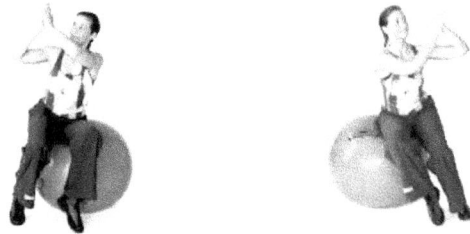

LIFT

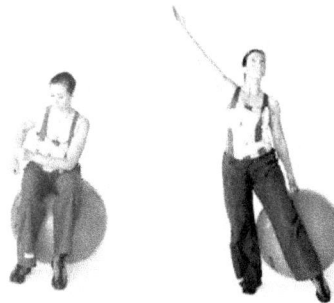

EXERCISE	NOTES	VARIATION
Sit on the ball. Torso erect. Bounce on the ball with the feet on the floor iniatially, then lifting off the floor. Dynamic arm movements.	Basic warm up exercise. Keep knees and feet aligned, no rotation of the knees. Contract the core, including the pelvic floor muscles, to stabilize.	Without arm movements. With various arm movements. With the eyes closed. Amplitude changes. Rhythm changes and hop combinations.
Sit on the ball. Torso erect. Bounce on the ball. Twist the hips and legs from side to side. Dynamic arm movements.	Basic warm up exercise. Keep knees and feet aligned, no rotation of the knees. Lift the heels, when twisting. Contract the core muscles, to stabilize.	Without arm movements. With various arm movements. Amplitude changes. Rhythm changes, eg. single/single/double twist.
Sit on the ball. Torso erect. Take a step to the side. Other foot steps together and makes a toe tap on the floor. Reverse, step back to the starting point. Dynamic arm movements.	Basic warm up exercise. Keep knees and feet aligned, no rotation of the knees. Contract the core muscles, to stabilize.	Without arm movements. With various arm movements. Single or double step. **SIDE ROLLING** From a double step, push off and roll to the side, while lifting feet off the floor in the middle part of the movement.
Sit on the ball. Torso erect. Take a step to the side. Stand up and lift the opposite leg. Put the hand on the ball to control it; keep it from rolling away. Sit down again, and step back to the starting point and lift.	Intermediate warm up exercise. Keep knees and feet aligned, no rotation of the knees. Contract the core muscles, to stabilize.	Without arm movements. With various arm movements. Lift leg into hip flexion, abduction or extension. Single or double step. Amplitude changes.

JAZZ SQUARE

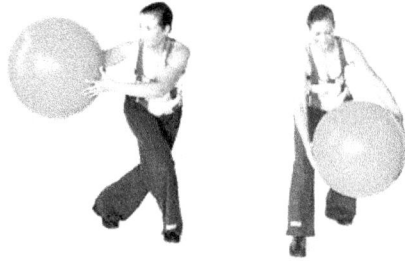

CHASSÉ

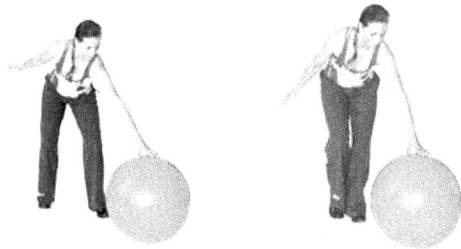

GRAPEVINE

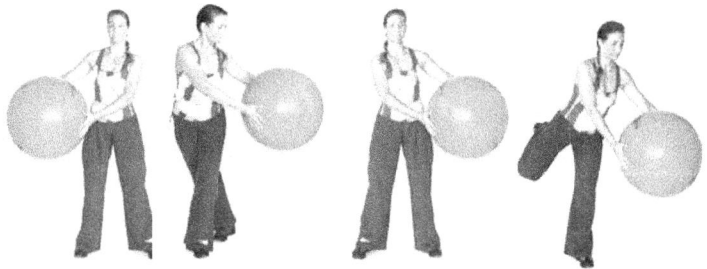

STEP TOUCH

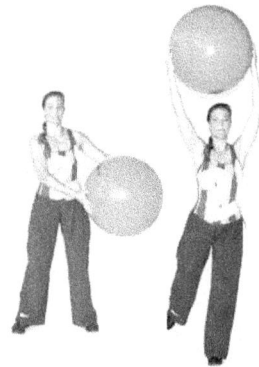

Walking step: Jazz step, jazz square or box step: Four-part walking step: You cross the foot over at the first or the second walking step and then walk to step back. Hands hold the ball. Make circling movements with the ball.	Low impact movement, which can be stylized to become more 'jazzy'.	Without arm movements. With various arm movements. Walk forward, cross over, step back, step back. Or: Cross over, step back, step back, walk forward.
Walking-sliding movement: Three quick steps to the side on the count of "1-and-2" (often counted as 1-2-3). Control the ball with the hand.	Low impact movement, which can be stylized to become more 'jazzy' or 'latin'.	Without arm movements. With various arm movements. Carry the ball or roll the ball. Chassé forward, backward, to the side or in circles.
Four-part walking step: Step to the side, cross behind, step out, feet together – or a tap or leg lift. Stay and do something else or return to the starting point.	Popular low impact movement. Perform the movement right and left – and also left and right, as this provides variety and a balanced workout.	Without arm movements. With various arm movements. Carry the ball or roll the ball. Cross in front of the opposite leg. Tempo or rhythm changes.
Two-part walking step: Step to the side, follow and tap or lift the opposite foot/leg. Stay and do something else or return to the starting point.	Popular low impact movement. Perform the movement right and left – and also left and right, as this provides variety and a balanced workout.	Without arm movements. With various arm movements. Carry, roll or bounce the ball. Tempo or rhythm changes. Step 1, 2, 3 or 4 steps to the side – or forward.

WALK	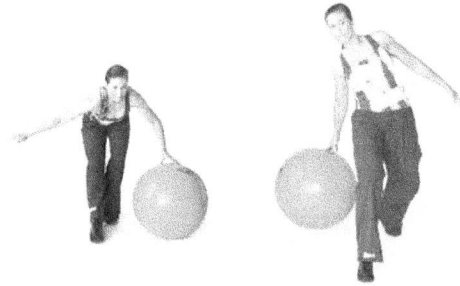
STEP (HAMSTRING) CURL	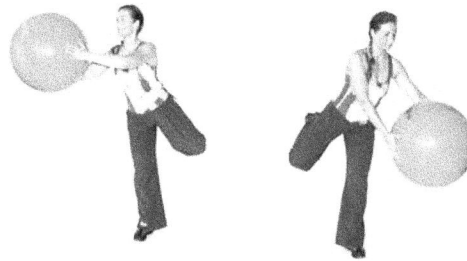
SKIP	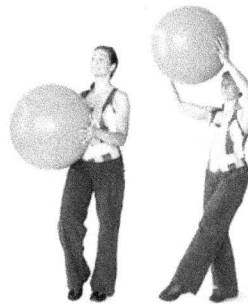
KNEELIFT	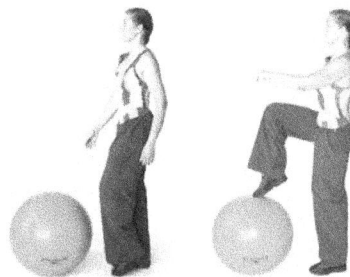

Walk. On the spot or in patterns. Hands hold, roll or bounce the ball.	Most low impact combinations come from walking. You can make endless variations.	Without arm movements. With various arm movements. Carry, roll or bounce the ball. Tempo or rhythm changes. Walk forward, backward, to the side, diagonally or in circles.
Step to the side, follow and bend the leg to perform a hamstring curl. Stay and repeat the curl or return to the starting point.	Popular low impact movement. Perform the movement right and left – and also left and right, as this provides variety and a balanced workout.	Without arm movements. With various arm movements. Carry, roll or bounce the ball. Tempo or rhythm changes, eg. single, single, double or repeaters 3, 4, 5, 6, 7.
Extend the knee and plantarflex the ankle, point the toes down. Make a small skip. On the spot or travelling.	Basic low impact movement, may also be performed in high impact.	Without arm movements. With various arm movements. Skip forward, to the side or backward. Tempo or rhythm changes, eg. single, single, double or repeaters 3, 4, 5, 6, 7.
Bend the hip and the knee. Lift the knee above horizontal. Hold the ball in the hands or control the ball with the feet, tap on top with left and right foot alternating.	Basic low impact move, may also be performed in high impact.	Without arm movements. With various arm movements. Kneelift forward, to the side or in front of other leg (crossover). Tempo or rhythm changes, eg. single, single, double or repeaters 3, 4, 5, 6, 7.

KICK

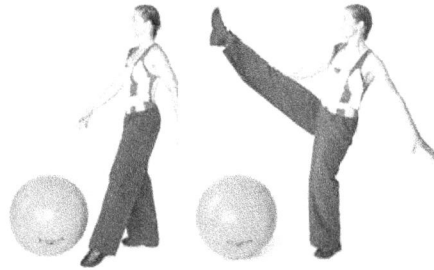

TWIST

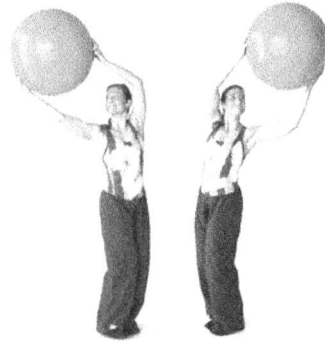

STEP OUT JACK

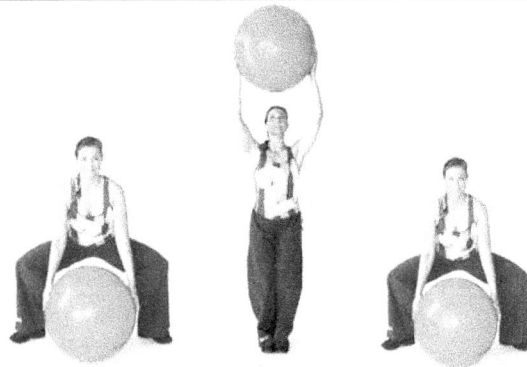

LUNGE

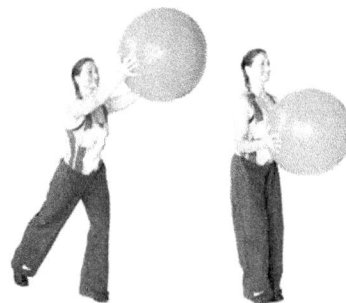

		VARIATIONS
Flex the hip, lift the leg. Keep the knee straight, when lifting and lowering. Ball on the floor or in the hands.	Basic low impact move, may also be performed in high impact.	Without arm movements. With various arm movements. Kick forward, to the side or backward (extension). Or swing leg over the ball in a semi-circular movement. Tempo or rhythm changes, eg. single, single, double or repeaters 3, 4, 5, 6, 7.
Raise the heels, get up on the toes, twist the hips and legs from side to side. Hold the ball in the hands.	Basic low impact move, may also be performed in high impact.	Without arm movements. With various arm movements. Tempo or rhythm changes, eg. single, single, double or repeaters 3, 4, 5.
Feet together. Take a large step to the side and bend both legs, bodyweight centered between the legs. Push off and step back, adduct the legs. Repeat or repeat to the opposite side.	Basic low impact move, it is the low impact variation of jumping jacks (high impact).	Without arm movements. With various arm movements. Amplitude and tempo changes.
Standing, feet together. Push one leg straight back into (aerobic) lunge position. Bodyweight is centered over the front, bent, leg. Back leg is non-weightbearing and normally you only touch the toes to the floor. Repeat or repeat with the other leg.	Watch your achilles tendon: Small range of motion, and moderate tempo, lower the heel to the floor. Large range of motion, touch only the toes – do not lower the heel.	Without arm movements. With various arm movements.

5 | Upper Body Exercises

In this section you find upper body exercises, for the shoulders, chest, upper back and arms, with the stability ball, for one exerciser and in most cases with one ball – only a couple of exercises involve two balls. In most of the exercises you also work the core muscles – one of the major benefits of stability ball training.

The exercises are categorized after primary muscles and muscle groups and roughly 'from top to toe', not necessarily in the recommended sequence for a workout.

There is a wide selection of exercises and you have to make your own decision as to which exercise is better for your purpose.

Some exercises are very easy, some very difficult. In some cases there is a note telling, if it is an easy or difficult exercise, but not in all cases as many factors play a role. Some knowledge of sports science is necessary in order to be able to select the right exercise for a given exerciser.

Most exercises can be varied by using one or both arms or legs and changing the arm-, body- or leg-position.

The point of support can be changed, eg. from the hips to the thighs, to the lower legs, ankles or toes. This results in a marked increase of the load on the working muscles.

Most exercises can be made more difficult by decreasing the base of support, eg. from sitting on the ball with the feet wide apart to sitting with the feet together or just one foot on the floor.

Important: All exercises are for healthy exercisers free from any serious or disabilitating disease, illness or ailments. Please consult your doctor before beginning these exercises.

Muscles

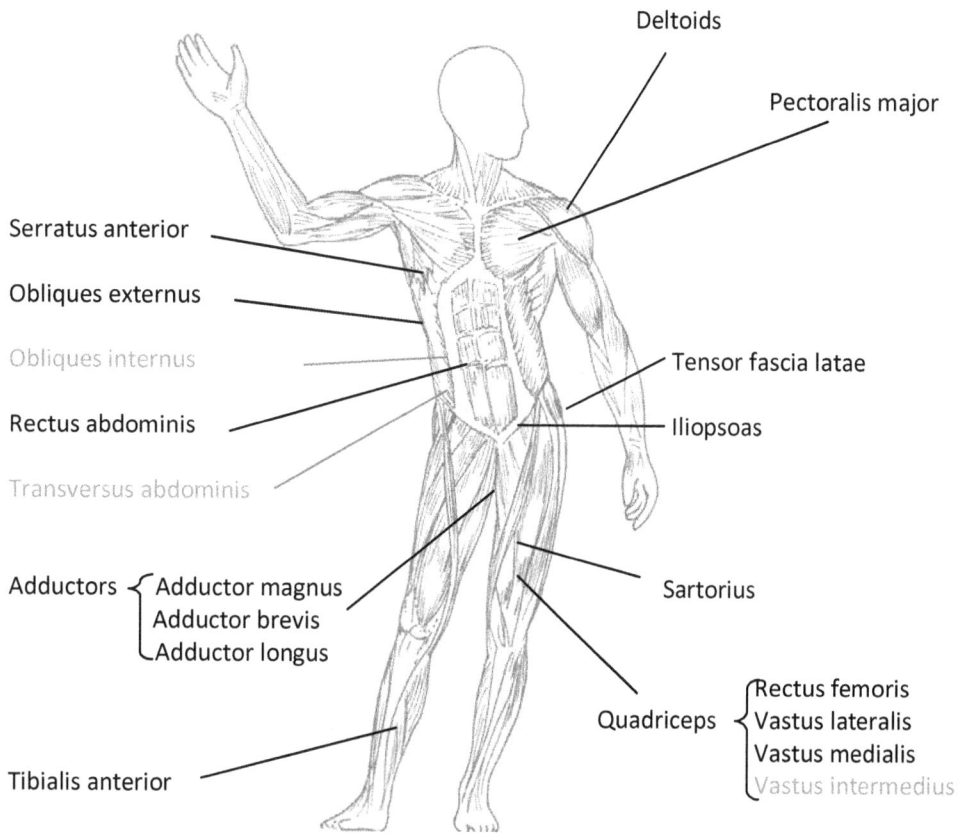

Deltoids

Pectoralis major

Serratus anterior

Obliques externus

Obliques internus

Rectus abdominis

Transversus abdominis

Tensor fascia latae

Iliopsoas

Adductors { Adductor magnus
Adductor brevis
Adductor longus

Sartorius

Quadriceps { Rectus femoris
Vastus lateralis
Vastus medialis
Vastus intermedius

Tibialis anterior

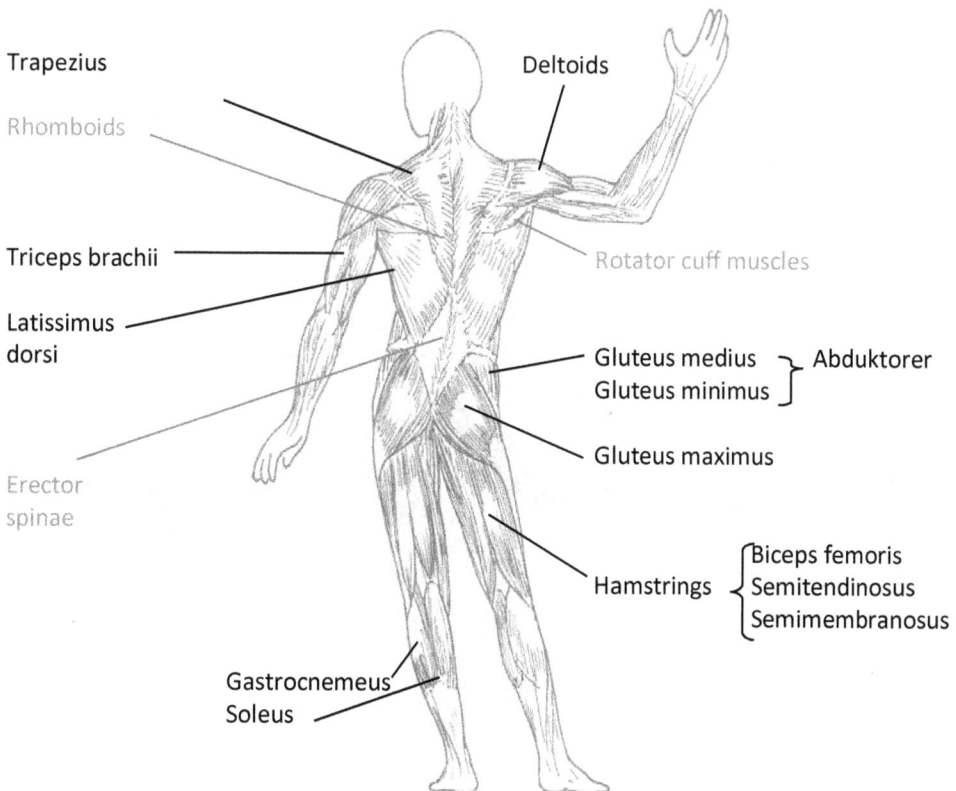

Trapezius

Rhomboids

Deltoids

Triceps brachii

Latissimus
dorsi

Rotator cuff muscles

Erector
spinae

Gluteus medius ⌐ Abduktorer
Gluteus minimus ⌡

Gluteus maximus

Biceps femoris
Hamstrings { Semitendinosus
Semimembranosus

Gastrocnemeus
Soleus

CHEST PUSH-UP
KNEELING ON FLOOR,
WITH HIP FLEXION

Primary muscles:
Pectoralis major, triceps
brachii, anterior deltoid

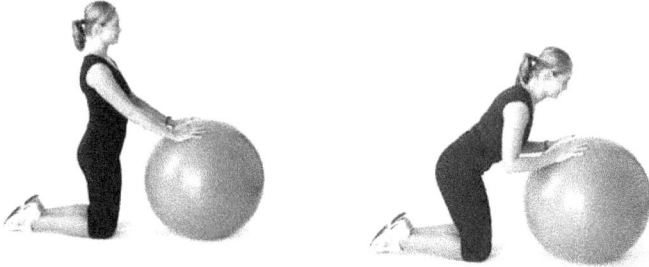

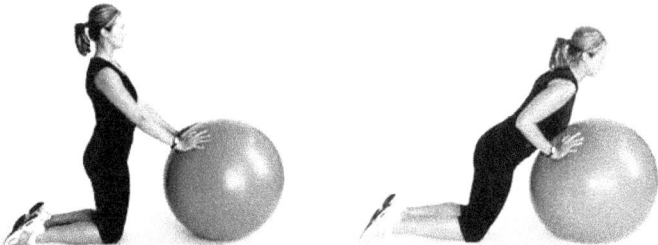

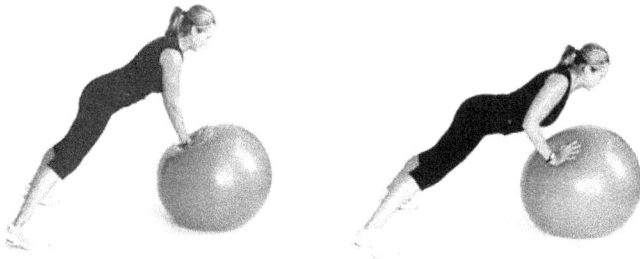

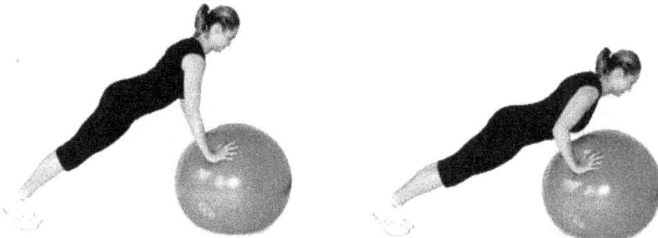

CHEST PUSH-UP
KNEELING
ON THE FLOOR

Primary muscles:
Pectoralis major, triceps
brachii, anterior deltoid

CHEST PUSH-UP
PLANK POSITION
LEGS WIDE ON THE FLOOR

Primary muscles:
Pectoralis major, triceps
brachii, anterior deltoid

CHEST PUSH-UP
PLANK POSITION
HANDS ON THE BALL

Primary muscles:
Pectoralis major, triceps
brachii, anterior deltoid

Kneeling on floor behind ball. Thighs close to the ball. Torso erect. The hands wide on ball, fingers forward/outward. Bend the arms, so the torso is lowered down towards the ball. Extend the arms, push the body back up again.	Easy exercise, suitable for novices and beginners. Keep the neck, shoulder girdle and the lower back in neutral position throughout the exercise. Avoid locking, hyperextending, the elbows in top position.	Different arm/leg position.
Kneeling on the floor behind the ball. Hands wide on the ball, forward and outward. Contract the core muscles. Bend the arms, so the body is lowered down towards the ball. Extend the arms, push the body back up again.	Keep the neck, shoulder girdle and the lower back in neutral position throughout the exercise. Avoid locking, hyperextending, the elbows in top position.	Different arm/leg position.
Plank position. Hands on top of the ball. Feet wide apart on the floor. Contract the core muscles. Bend the arms, so the body is lowered down towards the ball. Extend the arms, push the body back up again.	Neck, shoulder girdle and lower back in neutral position throughout the exercise. Avoid locking, hyperextending, the elbows in top position. This exercise may be hard on the wrists. They should be strengthened gradually; fewer repetitions in the beginning and mor rest between sets.	Different arm/body/leg position. Feet wide apart or together (easy or hard). Legs/feet may support on a bench, so the exercise becomes harder. Legs/feet may support on a balll, so extra balance work is added to the exercise.
Plank position. Hands wide on the ball, forward and outward. Feet on the floor, together or hip-width apart. Contract the core muscles. Bend the arms, so the body is lowered towards the ball. Extend the arms, push the body back up again.	Neck, shoulder girdle and lower back in neutral position throughout the exercise. Avoid locking, hyperextending, the elbows in top position. This exercise may be hard on the wrists. They should be strengthened gradually; fewer repetitions in the beginning and more rest between sets.	Different arm/body/leg position. Support on one or both legs. **ROTATED PUSH-UP** Rotate the ball and body slightly to the side. Perform a push-up. Repeat to the other side.

CHEST PUSH-UP
PLANK POSITION
THIGHS ON THE BALL

Primary muscles:
Pectoralis major, triceps
brachii, anterior deltoid

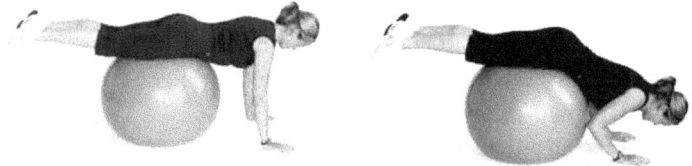

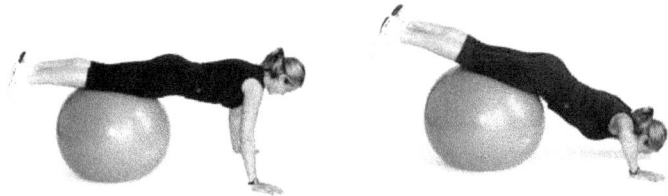

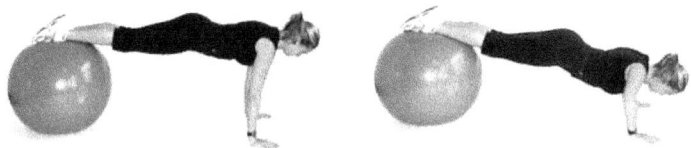

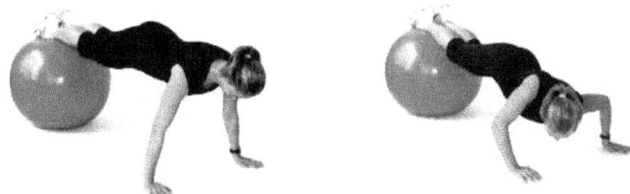

CHEST PUSH-UP
PLANK POSITION
THIGHS ON THE BALL

Primary muscles:
Pectoralis major, triceps
brachii, anterior deltoid

CHEST PUSH-UP
PLANK POSITION
LOWER LEGS ON THE BALL

Primary muscles:
Pectoralis major, triceps
brachii, anterior deltoid

LATERAL CHEST PUSH-UP
PLANK POSITION
LOWER LEGS ON THE BALL

Primary muscles:
Pectoralis major, triceps
brachii, anterior deltoid

Plank position. Hips on top of the ball. Hands wide apart on the floor. Contract the core muscles. Bend the arms, so the body is lowered down towards the floor. Extend the arms, push the body back up again.	Neck, shoulder girdle and lower back in neutral position throughout the exercise. Avoid locking, hyperextending, the elbows in top position. This position may be hard on the wrists. They should be strengthened gradually; fewer repetitions in the beginning and more rest between sets.	Different arm/leg position. **POWER PUSH** From push-up position push off with the arms, roll backwards and sit down behind the ball. Push off with the legs and roll back forward to push-up position.
Plank position. Thighs on top of the ball. Hands wide apart on the floor. Contract the core muscles. Bend the arms and lower the body down towards the floor. Extend the arms, push the body back up again.	Neck, shoulder girdle and lower back in neutral position throughout the exercise. Avoid locking, hyperextending, the elbows in top position. This position may be hard on the wrists. They should be strengthened gradually; fewer repetitions in the beginning and more rest between sets.	Different arm/leg position. **ASYMMETRICAL PUSH-UP** One hand in front of the other. Perform a push-up. After a set repeat with the opposite hand in front. Or you may alternate between each push-up.
Plank position. Lower legs on top of the ball. Hands wide apart on the floor. Contract the core muscles. Bend the arms and lower the body down towards the floor. Extend the arms, push the body back up again.	Neck, shoulder girdle and lower back in neutral position throughout the exercise. Avoid locking, hyperextending, the elbows in top position. This position may be hard on the wrists. They should be strengthened gradually; fewer repetitions in the beginning and more rest between sets.	Different arm/leg position. Legs may rotate to one side to a slightly rotated hip- and body position. **EXPLOSIVE PUSH-UP** Push off forcefully with the arms; hands off the floor. Land on hands with control.
Plank position. Lower legs on top of the ball. Hands wide apart on the floor. Contract the core muscles. Bend the arms and lower the body down and to one side, lateral push-up. Extend the arms, push the body back up again. Repeat to the other side.	The neck, shoulder girdle and lower back in neutral position throughout the exercise. Avoid locking, hyperextending, the elbows in top position. This position may be hard on the wrists. They should be strengthened gradually; fewer repetitions in the beginning and more rest between sets.	Different arm/body/leg position. Support on hips, thighs, lower legs or toes (easy to hard). **PUSH-UP WITH HIP ROTATION** Push-up straight up and down. During the push-up rotate hips and legs from side to the side.

**WALK WITH HANDS AND
FEET WIDE APART
PRONE ON THE BALL**

Primary muscles:
Pectoralis major, anterior and
posterior deltoid, transversus
abdominis, multifidii

**PLANK
ARM 'WALKING' NARROW
PLANK POSITION**

Primary muscles:
Pectoralis major, latissimus
dorsi, deltoids, transversus
abdominis, multifidii

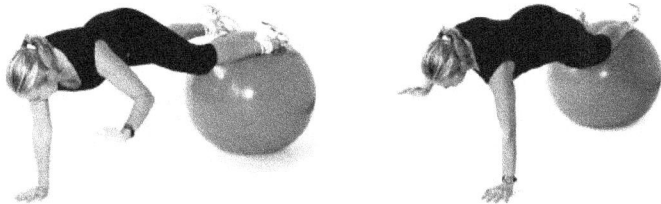

**CHEST/ARM PULL,
SIDE TO SIDE
PLANK POSITION**

Primary muscles:
Pectoralis major, biceps
brachii, anterior deltoid,
transversus abd., multifidii

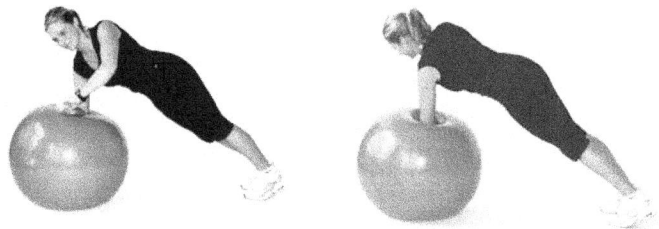

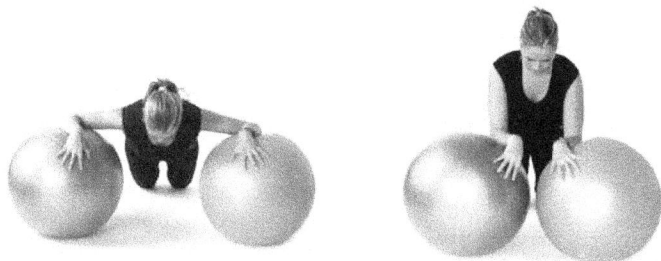

**CHEST FLY, TWO BALLS
DUAL BALL FLY
PLANK POSITION**

Primary muscles:
Pectoralis major,
anterior deltoid,
transversus abd., multifidii

Prone on the ball. Arms and legs wide apart. Walk with the right arm and the right leg on the floor, the body rolls tilts to the right. Alternate. Walk with the left arm and left leg on the floor, the body tilts to the left. Dynamic movement from side to side.	Neck, shoulder girdle and lower back in neutral position throughout the exercise. Contract the core muscles to stabilize. Contract the thigh muscles to protect the knees.	Range of motion. More or less force. Slower or faster movement.
Plank position. The hips or legs on the ball. The hands on the floor under the shoulders, arms vertical, body is kept steady. Walk with the hands. Pull the elbows upwards closely past the torso towards the ceiling. Contract the core muscles to stabilize the body.	Neck, shoulder girdle and lower back in neutral position throughout the exercise. Contract the core muscles to stabilize.	Different arm/leg position. Support on the hips, the thighs, lower legs or the toes (easy to hard).
Sideplank position. Feet on the floor. Elbows bent 90 degrees, hands together. One forearm on the ball, other forearm vertical. Pull the other forearm down and into the ball, so the arms change position on the stability ball. Alternate.	Neck, shoulder girdle and lower back in neutral position throughout the exercise. Contract the core muscles to stabilize.	Different body/leg position. Feet wide apart or together (easy to hard).
Kneeling behind the ball. The elbows are bent 90 degr. One forearm on each ball. Upper arms to the side, close to horizontal. Contract the chest muscles and pull the arms inwards, so the balls are pulled towards each other. Return the arms to the sides, resisting the movement.	For advanced exercisers. Requires strength and stabilty. Avoid lowering the body too much, as this is hard on the shoulders (ligaments). Neck, shoulder girdle and lower back in neutral position. Contract the core muscles to stabilize.	Different body/leg position. By bending the hips, the exercise becomes easier. Can be performed in plank position with the toes on the floor (for advanced exercisers).

**CHEST SQUEEZE
STANDING ON THE FLOOR**

Primary muscles:
Pectoralis major,
anterior deltoid,
biceps brachii

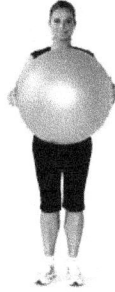

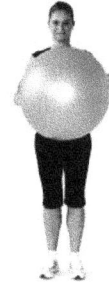

**SHOULDER BLADE SQUEEZE
STANDING ON THE FLOOR**

Primary muscles:
Rhomboids,
Trapezius, medial part

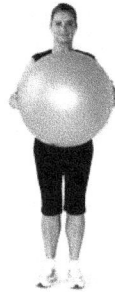

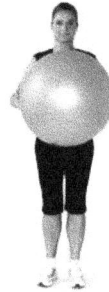

**SHRUGS
WITH BALL OVERHEAD
SITTING ON THE FLOOR**

Primary muscles:
Trapezius, levator scapulae

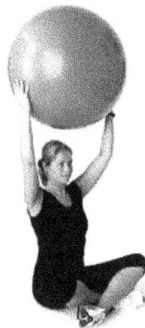

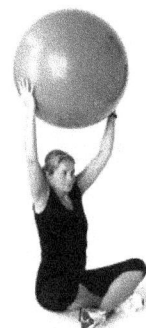

**BOXING MOTION
BRIDGE POSITION**

Primary muscles: Pectoralis
major, rhomboids, deltoids,
arm muscles, gluteus maximus,
hamstrings, obliques,
transversus abd., multifidii

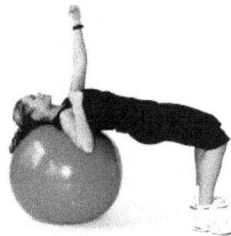

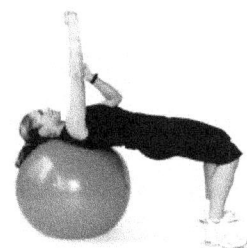

Standing on the floor. Hands on each side of the ball. Contract the chest muscles and push the hands into the stability ball, as if to squeeze it out of shape. Isometric or dynamic.	Remember to keep breathing.	Different arm/body/leg position. Standing, kneeling, sitting, supine.
Standing on the floor. Hands on each side of the ball. Contract the muscles between the shoulder blades, adduct the shoulder blades. Move the shoulder blades away from each other, back to neutral position.	Easy basic exercise. In this position there is no direct load on these muscles. The exercise is for mobilization. Keep the neck and the spine in neutral position throughout the exercise. Contract the core muscles to stabilize.	Different leg position. Standing, kneeling, sitting, supine.
Sitting on the floor. The hands hold the ball. The arms are extended over the head. No movement in the elbows. Lift the shoulders and the ball with the upper back (and neck) muscles. Lower with control.	Easy exercise. For added resistance use a medicine ball. Keep the neck and the spine in neutral position throughout the exercise. Contract the core muscles to stabilize.	Different arm/leg position. Standing, kneeling, sitting. Sitting on a stability ball. For more core work the arms can be held forward at a 45 degree angle to the torso.
Bridge position. Shoulder blades on the ball. Feet on the floor. The arms are vertical. Make a boxing movement, towards the ceiling, with the right and left arm alternating. Contract the obliques to rotate the torso at the same time.	Keep the neck and the spine in neutral position throughout the exercise. Contract the core muscles to stabilize. Create resistance by pressing the torso into the ball. A dynamic exercise.	Different leg position. Legs wide apart or together (easy or hard).

SERRATUS PRESS (SCAPULAR PRESS) SUPINE ON THE BALL Primary muscles: Rhomboids, Trapezius, medial part, serratus	
SERRATUS PUSH-UP (SCAPULAR PUSH-UP) PLANK POSITION THIGHS ON THE BALL Primary muscles: Subscapularis, serratus anterior	
SERRATUS PUSH-UP (SCAPULAR PUSH-UP) PLANK POSITION LOWER LEG ON THE BALL Primary muscles: Subscapularis, serratus anterior	
SERRATUS PUSH-UP (SCAPULAR PUSH-UP) PLANK POSITION HANDS ON THE BALL Primary muscles: Subscapularis, serratus anterior	

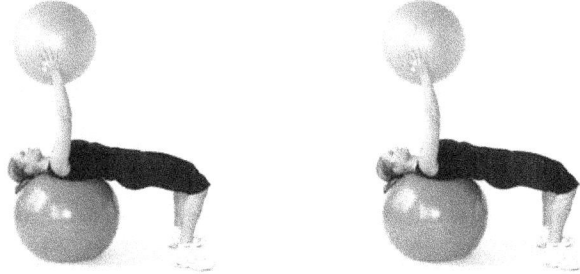

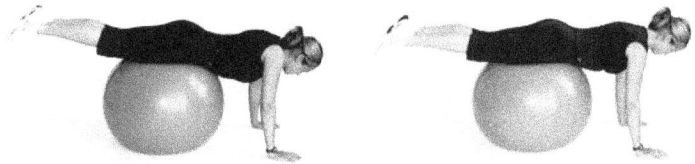

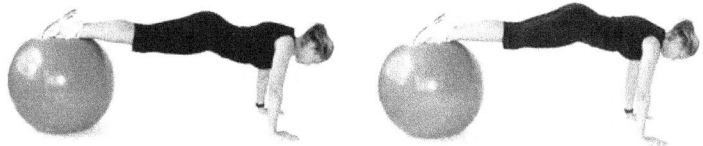

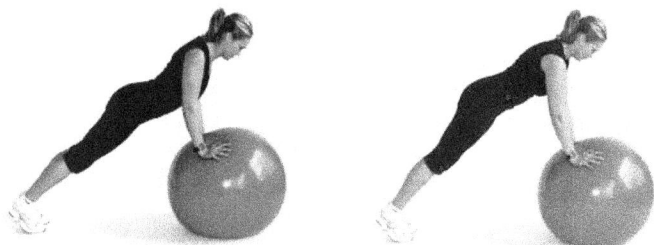

Supine. Shoulder blades on the ball. Buttocks contract to keep the body in bridge position. Arms in vertical position, ball in the hands. Adduct the shoulder blades and release back to neutral position. Press into the ball for added resistance.	Neck and spine in neutral throughout the exercise. Contract the core muscles to stabilize. The arms are kept straight throughout the exercise, it is a shoulder blade movement.	Different leg position. With or without a ball in the hands. With a medicine ball.
Plank position. Hands on the floor. Hips on the ball. The arms are kept straight, no movement in the elbows. Contract and abduct, retract the shoulder blades. Return. Resist movement as the shoulder blades return to neutral.	Neck and spine in neutral throughout the exercise. Contract the core muscles to stabilize. The arms are kept straight throughout the exercise, it is a shoulder blade movement.	Different arm/leg position.
Plank position. Hands on the floor. Feet on the ball. The arms are kept straight, no movement in the elbows. Contract and abduct, retract the shoulder blades. Return. Resist movement as the shoulder blades return to neutral.	Neck, shoulder girdle and the lower back in neutral throughout the exercise. Contract the core muscles to stabilize. The arms are kept straight throughout the exercise, it is a shoulder blade movement.	Different arm/leg position.
Plank position. Hands on the ball. Feet on the floor. The arms are kept straight, no movement in the elbows. Contract and abduct, retract the shoulder blades. Return. Resist movement as the shoulder blades return to neutral.	Neck, shoulder girdle and the lower back in neutral throughout the exercise. Contract the core muscles to stabilize. The arms are kept straight throughout the exercise, it is a shoulder blade movement.	Different arm/body/leg position. Legs wide apart (easier). On one leg (added balance work).

**TRICEPS DIPS
HANDS ON THE BALL**

Primary muscles:
Triceps brachii, deltoids

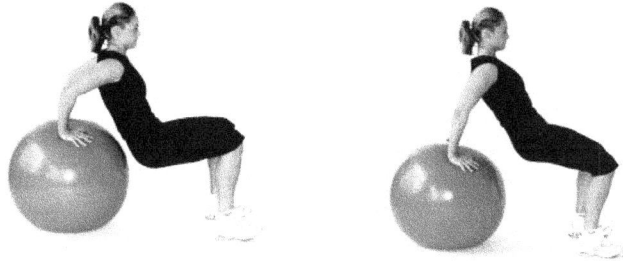

**TRICEPS PUSH-UP
PLANK POSITION
HIPS ON THE BALL**

Primary muscles:
Triceps brachii, deltoids,
pectoralis major

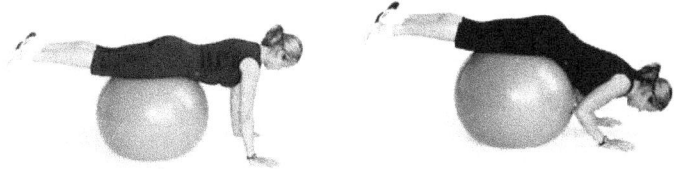

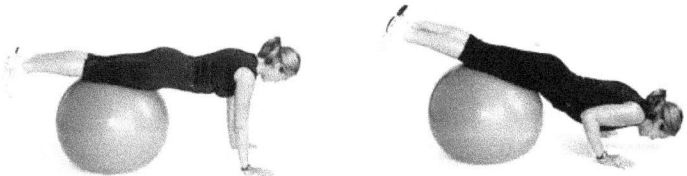

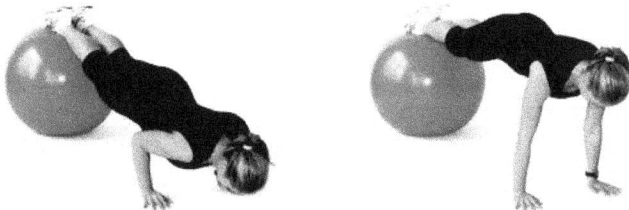

**TRICEPS PUSH-UP
PLANK POSITION
THIGHS ON THE BALL**

Primary muscles:
Triceps brachii, deltoids,
pectoralis major

**TRICEPS PUSH-UP
PLANK POSITION
LOWER LEGS ON THE BALL**

Primary muscles:
Triceps brachii, deltoids,
pectoralis major

Bridge position. Back to the ball. Hands on the ball, the fingers point forward toward the body. Feet on the floor. Bend the arms, so the buttocks are lowered down towards the floor close to the ball. Keep the shoulders lowered throughout the exercise. Return. Extend the arms.	Challnging exercise for the shoulder girdle (and balance). Initially perform smaller movements at moderate tempo. Contract the core muscles to stabilize. Avoid locking, hyperextending, the elbows in top position.	Different body/leg position. Legs bent or straight.
Plank position. Hips on the ball. Hands shoulder-width apart on the floor. Bend the arms, the elbows move straight backwards, and lower the body down towards the floor. Return. Extend the arms.	Neck, shoulder girdle and lower back in neutral position throughout the exercise. Contract the core muscles to stabilize. Avoid locking, hyperextending, the elbows in top position.	Different arm/leg position. Hands together and elbows out. Hands shoulder-width apart and hinge push up (forearms to the floor and up).
Plank position. Thighs on the ball. Hands shoulder-width apart on the floor. Bend the arms, the elbows move straight backwards, lower the body ned towards the floor. Return. Extend the arms.	Neck, shoulder girdle and lower back in neutral position. Contract the core muscles to stabilize. Avoid locking, hyperextending, the elbows in top position.	Different arm/leg position. Hands together and elbows out. Hands shoulder-width apart and hinge push up (forearms to the floor and back up).
Plank position. Toes or lower legs on the ball. Hands shoulder-width apart on the floor. Bend the arms, the elbows move straight back, and lower the body down towards the floor. Return. Extend the arms.	For advanced exercisers. Neck, shoulder girdle and lower back in neutral position. Contract the core muscles to stabilize. Avoid locking, hyperextending, the elbows in top position.	Different arm/leg position. Hands together, elbows out. Hands shoulder-width apart and hinge push up (forearms to the floor and back up). **EXPLOSIVE PUSH-UP** From this position arms push off explosively, so the body is propelled upwards, hands off the floor (advanced exercisee).

TRICEPS PUSH-UP
PLANK POSITION
ONE LEG ON THE BALL

Primary muscles:
Triceps brachii, deltoids,
pectoralis major

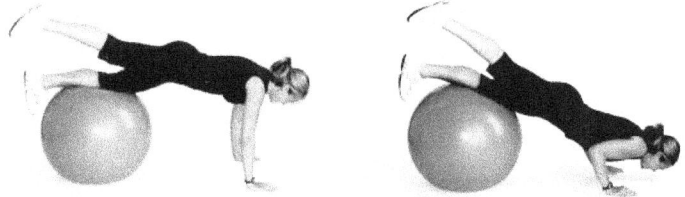

TRICEPS PUSH-UP
HANDS TOGETHER
PLANK POSITION
FEET ON THE BALL

Primary muscles:
Triceps brachii,
anterior deltoids

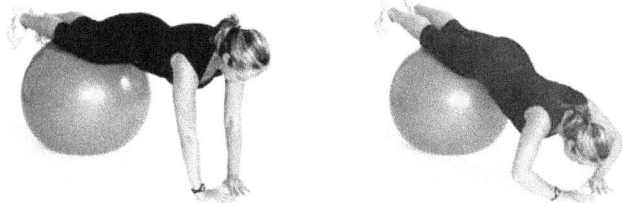

SHOULDER/TRICEPS PRESS
(TUCK SHOULDER PRESS)
KNEELING ON THE BALL

Primary muscles:
Triceps brachii,
anterior and medial deltoids

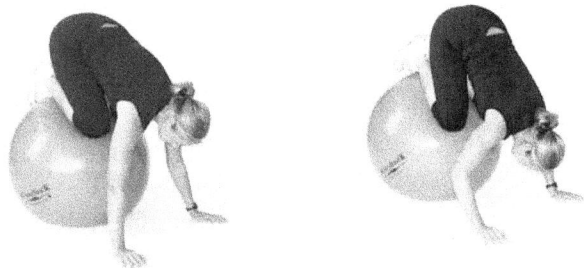

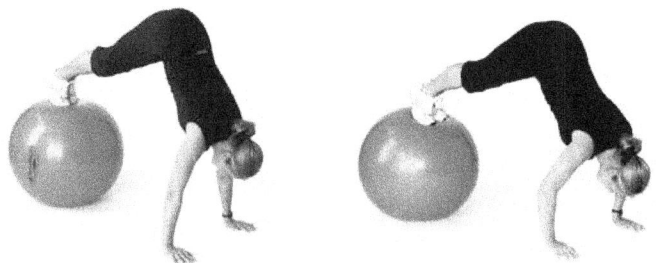

SHOULDER/TRICEPS PRESS
(PIKE SHOULDER PRESS)
PLANK POSITION
TOES ON THE BALL

Primary muscles:
Triceps brachii,
anterior and medial deltoids

Plank position. One thigh on the ball, the other leg is lifted off the ball. Keep the pelvis level, stable. Hands shoulder-width apart on the floor. Bend the arms, the elbows move straight backwards, and lower the body down towards the floor. Return.	For advanced exercisers. Neck, shoulder girdle and lower back in neutral position. Contract the core muscles to stabilize. Avoid locking, hyperextending, the elbows in top position.	Different arm/leg position. Hands together and elbows out. Hands shoulder-width apart and hinge push up (forearms to the floor and back up).
Plank position. Thighs or lower legs on the ball. Hands on the floor. Index fingers and thumbs together. Bend the arms, the elbows move diagonally backwards, and lower the body down towards the floor. Return. Extend the arms.	For advanced exercisers. Neck, shoulder girdle and lower back in neutral position. Contract the core muscles to stabilize. Avoid locking, hyperextending, the elbows in top position.	Support on the hips, the thighs, lower legs or the toes (easy to hard).
Plank position. Lower legs on the ball. Hands shoulder-width or wider apart on the floor. The body is 'crunching' on top of the ball. Bend the arms and lower the torso down towards the floor. Return. Push off with the arms and shoulders.	For advanced exercisers Neck, shoulder girdle and lower back in neutral position. Contract the core muscles to stabilize. Avoid locking, hyperextending, the elbows in top position.	Different arm/leg position.
Plank position. Feet on the ball. Legs straight. Hips flexed. The body in pike position on the ball. Hands wide apart, more than shoulder-width apart, on the floor. Bend the arms and lower the body down towards the floor. Extend the arms.	For very advanced exercisers Neck, shoulder girdle and lower back in neutral position. Contract the core muscles to stabilize. Avoid locking, hyperextending, the elbows in top position.	Different arm/leg position. **PIKE PRESS ON ONE LEG** Same exercise, but only on one leg (very advanced exercise) (Juan Carlos Santana).

TRICEPS PUSH-UP
KNEELING ON THE FLOOR

Primary muscles:
Pectoralis major,
triceps brachii,
anterior deltoid

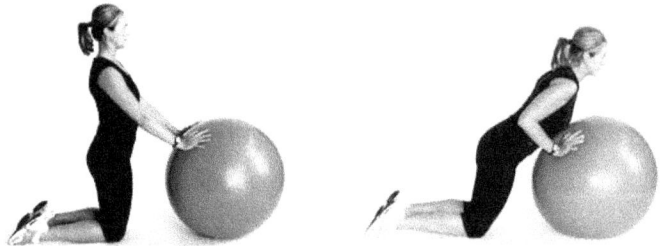

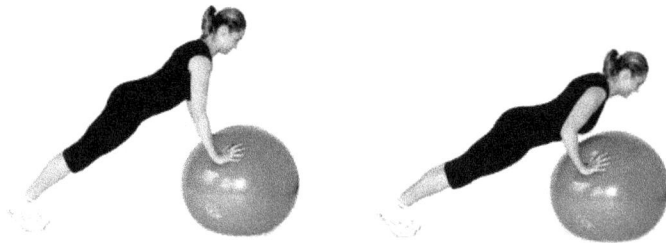

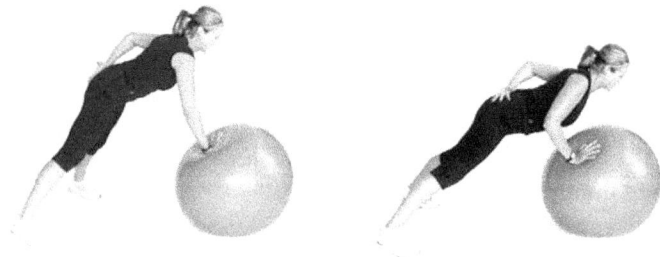

TRICEPS PUSH-UP
PLANK POSITION
HANDS ON THE BALL

Primary muscles:
Pectoralis major,
triceps brachii,
anterior deltoid

TRICEPS 1-ARM PUSH-UP
PLANK POSITION
ONE HAND ON THE BALL

Primary muscles:
Pectoralis major, triceps
brachii, anterior deltoid

TRICEPS PUSH-UP
WITH LAT PULL AND CIRCLE
PRONE ON THE BALL

Primary muscles: Triceps
brachii, deltoids, latissimus
dorsi, transversus abdominis,
multifidii

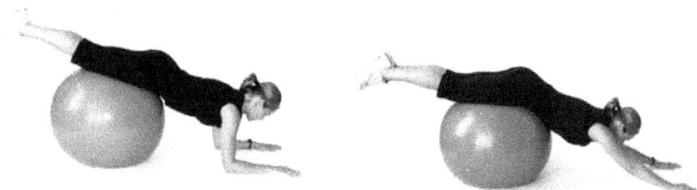

Kneeling on the floor behind the ball. Hands shoulder-width apart on the ball, elbows straight back. Contract the core muscles. Bend the arms, so the body is lowered down towards the ball. Extend the arms, push the body back up again.	For begining exercisers. Neck, shoulder girdle and lower back in neutral position throughout the exercise. Avoid locking, hyperextending, the elbows in top position.	Different arm/leg position.
Plank position. Hands on the ball, the elbows straight backward. Feet on the floor, together or hip-width apart. Contract the core muscles. Bend the arms, so the body lowers down towards the ball. Extend the arms, push the body back up again.	For advanced exercisers. Neck, shoulder girdle and lower back in neutral position throughout the exercise. Avoid locking, hyperextending, the elbows in top position.	Different arm/body/leg position. Feet wide apart or together (easier or harder). **STRADDLE PUSH-UP** Feet wide apart. Hands on the ball. Push-up.
Plank position. One hand centrered on the ball. Free arm forward, outward or backward. Feet on the floor, shoulder-width apart. Bend the arm, so the body is lowered down towards the ball. Extend the arm, push the body back up again.	For very advanced exercisers. Neck, shoulder girdle and lower back in neutral position. Avoid locking, hyperextending, the elbows in top position. Progression: Kneeling, standing feet wide apart, then feet shoulder-width apart.	Different arm/leg position.
Plank position. Thighs on the ball. Arms forward, hands on the floor. 1) Bend the arms so the body is lowered. 2) Pull the body forwards, the upper arms are pulled into the sides, roll forward on the stability ball. 3) Extend the arms up. 4) Push off with the arms, so the body and the ball roll backwards.	For intermediate exercisers. Neck, shoulder girdle and lower back in neutral position. Contract the core muscles to stabilize. You must be able to control all four phases of the exercise.	Support on the thighs or lower legs (hard). Reverse the sequence.

LAT PULL
WITH BACK EXTENSION
KNEELING ON THE FLOOR

Primary muscles:
Latissimus dorsi, posterior
deltoid, erector spinae,
transversus abdominis

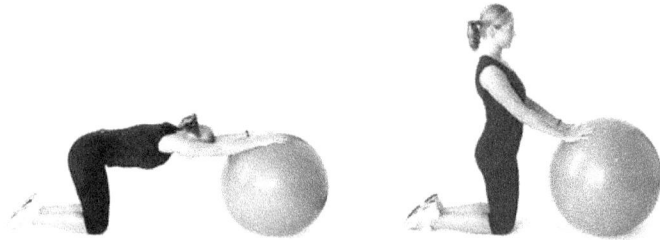

LAT PULL
KNEELING ON THE FLOOR

Primary muscles:
Latissimus dorsi, biceps brachii,
transversus abdominis,
multifidii

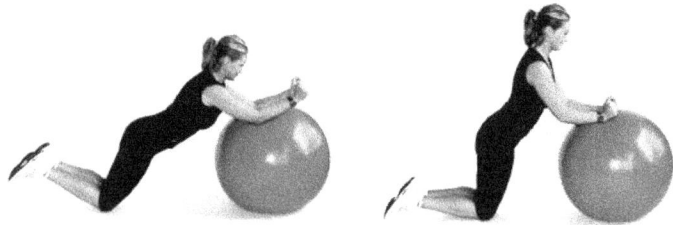

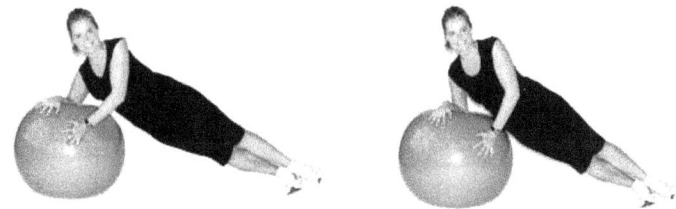

LAT PULL (LATERAL)
WITH THE BALL
SIDEPLANK POSITION

Primary muscles:
Latissimus dorsi, biceps brachii,
transversus abdominis,
multifidii

PULLOVER WITH THE BALL
BRIDGE POSITION
ON THE BALL

Primary muscles:
Latissimus dorsi,
pectoralis major,
gluteus maximus, hamstrings

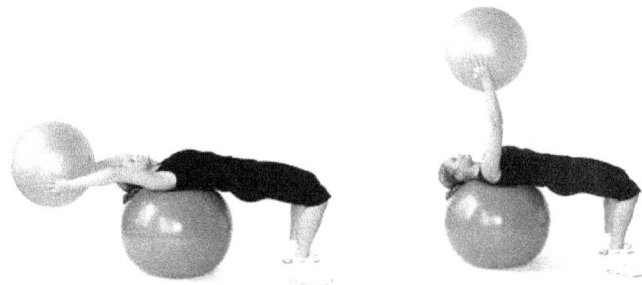

Kneeling behind the ball. Hands on the ball, shoulder-width apart or together. Push the arms into the ball and lean torso forward into horizontal position. Contract the back muscles and pull the arms back and close to the body, while returning to upright position.	Basic exercise, for beginners. Contract the core muscles to stabilize. Avoid using the hips and legs to move the body backward and forward. Use the back muscles.	Can be combined with other exercises in the end range of motion.
Kneeling behind the ball. Body in plank position with forearms on the ball with the hands together. Pull the arms back and close to the body, so the body returns to upright position. Return, move back into plank position with a controlled movement.	Contract the core muscles to stabilize. Advanced exercisers can roll out even further, onto the upper arms.	Different arm/body/leg position. **LAT PULL PLANK POSITION** Support on the toes, so the exercise is performed in a regular plank position (hard, for very advanced exercisers).
Sideplank position. One forearm on the ball. Other hand hold on to the ball to keep the balance. Feet on the floor, staggered. Contract the core muscles to stabilize. Pull forearm and ball closer to the side of the body. Return with control.	For advanced exercisers. Contract the core muscles to stabilize. Range of motion is limited in this exercise.	Different leg position. May be performed kneeling on the floor (easier version).
Bridge position. Shoulder blades on the ball. Feet on the floor Arms vertical with a stability ball in the hands. Lower the arms and the ball backwards, until the upper arms are close to the ears. Return arms to vertical.	Very easy exercise for the upper back and chest. Primarily for stability and mobility. Contract the core muscles to stabilize.	The ball in the hands can be replaced by a medicine ball or dumbbell to provide strength training. Supine or bridge position.

**REVERSE FLYS
(BACK FLYS)
BRIDGE POSITION**

Primary muscles: Gluteus
maximus, hamstrings,
transversus abdominis,
multifidii rhomboids, deltoids

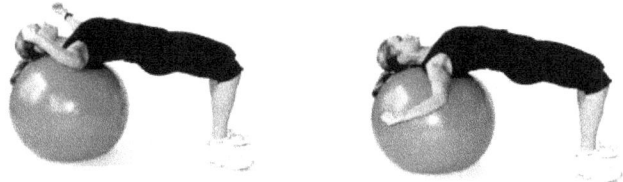

**REVERSE FLYS
PRONE ON THE BALL**

Primary muscles:
Rhomboids, erector spinae,
posterior deltoid,
transversus abdominis,
multifidii

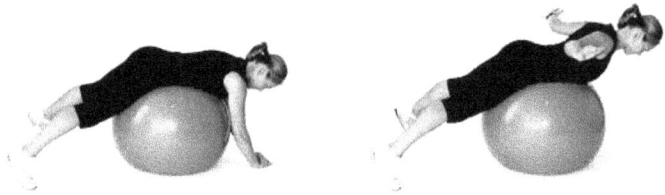

**LATERAL BALL ROLL
BRIDGE POSITION
HANDS ON THE BALL**

Primary muscles: Rhomboids,
deltoids, quadriceps, gluteus
maximus, hamstrings,
transversus abd., multifidii

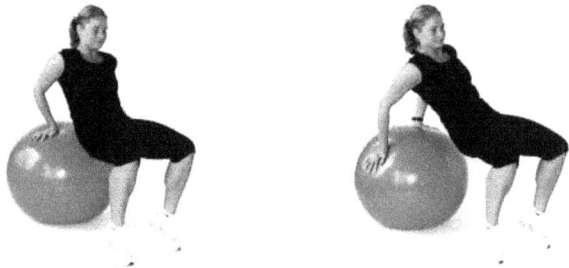

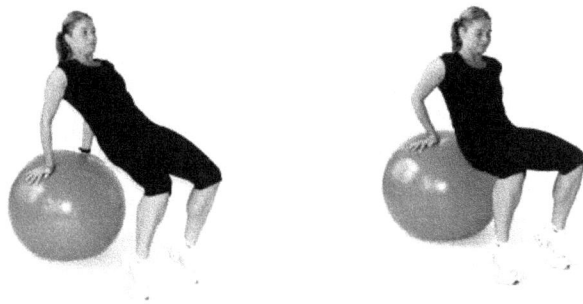

**SAGITTAL BALL PULL
BRIDGE POSITION
HANDS ON THE BALL**

Primary muscles:
Deltoids, quadriceps,
gluteus maximus, hamstrings,
transversus abd., multifidii

Supine with the shoulder blades on the ball. Feet on the floor, body in bridge position. Arms to the side. Contract the muscles between the shoulder blades. Pull the shoulder blades together and into the stability ball. Return to neutral.	Very easy exercise for the rhomboids. For increasing awareness of the muscles of the upper back. Contract the core muscles, the buttocks and the hamstrings to keep the bridge position.	Different leg position.
Prone on the ball. Feet on the floor. Contract the core muscles to stabilize. Keep the neck in neutral position. Arms down in front of the chest (ball) just above the floor. Lift the arms above horizontal and pull the shoulder blades together. Lower the arms.	Very easy rhomboid exercise. For learning the movement and increasing awareness of the muscles of the upper back. May be combined with back extension, when mastered. Contract the core muscles to stabilize.	Different leg/body position, with lower legs resting on the floor or with straight legs. Different arm position, diagonally forward, straight to the side, or diagonally back at various angles. Dumbbells in the hands for a strength training effect.
Bridge position, back to the ball. Hands on the ball, fingers point forward or outward. Feet on the floor, on the toes, the heels are lifted. Hold the position and roll the ball slightly from side to side.	For advanced exercisers. For shoulder stability. Can be hard on the shoulders and the wrists. Contract the core muscles to stabilize. Moderate tempo initially.	Different leg position.
Bridge position, back to the ball. Hands on the ball, fingers point forward or outward. Feet on the floor, on the toes, the heels are lifted. Hold the position and roll the ball slightly backward and forward.	For advanced exercisers. For shoulder stability. Can be hard on the shoulders and the wrists. Contract the core muscles to stabilize. Moderate tempo initially.	Different leg position.

6 | Core Exercises

In this section you find core exercises, for the outer and inner unit, abdominal muscles, back muscles and deep stabilizing muscles, with the stability ball, for one exerciser and one ball.

The exercises are categorized after primary muscles and muscle groups and not necessarily in the recommended sequence for a workout.

There is a wide selection of exercises and you have to make your own decision as to which exercise is better for your purpose.

Some exercises are very easy, some very difficult. In some cases there is a note to tell, if it is an easy or difficult exercise, but not in all cases as many factors play a role. Some knowledge of sports science is necessary in order to be able to select the right exercise for a given exerciser.

Most exercises can be varied by using one or both arms or legs and by changing the arm-, body- or leg position.

The point of support can be changed, eg. from the hips to the thighs, to the lower legs, ankles or toes. This results in a marked increase of the load on the muscles.

Most exercises can be made more difficult by increasing the balance work via decreasing the base of support, eg. from sitting on the ball with the feet wide apart to sitting with the feet together or just one foot on the floor.

Important: All exercises are for healthy exercisers free from any serious or disabilitating disease, illness or ailments. Please consult your doctor before beginning these exercises.

Core Muscles

Important core muscles are: The global (outer unit) muscles, the abdominal and back muscles, around the spine, the pelvic floor muscles, and the local (inner unit) muscles, a.o. the transversus abdominis and mm. multifidii, the 'corset muscles', which stabilizes the body.

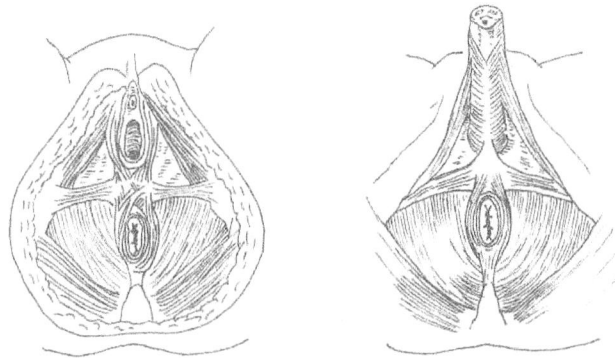

Pelvic floor muscles
Left: The female pelvic floor.
Right: The male pelvic floor.

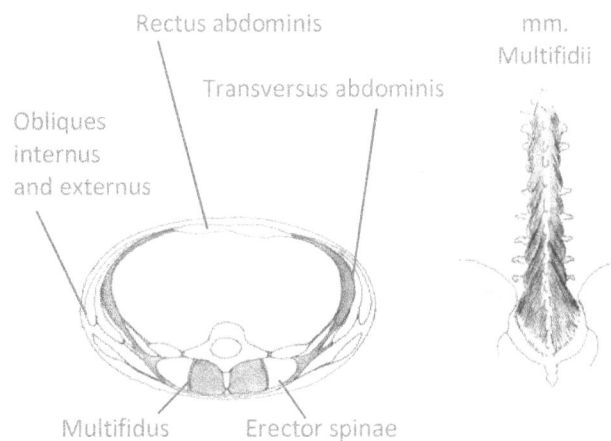

Left: A cross-section of the torso.
The spine is at the lower part of the drawing.
. The transversus abdominis and the mm. multifidii are accentuated by a darker colour.

Right: The mm. multifidii.

**AB CURL
SUPINE ON THE BALL**

Primary muscles:
Rectus abdominis,
obliques externus and
internus,
transversus abdominis

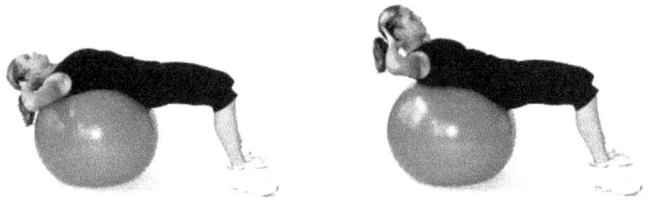

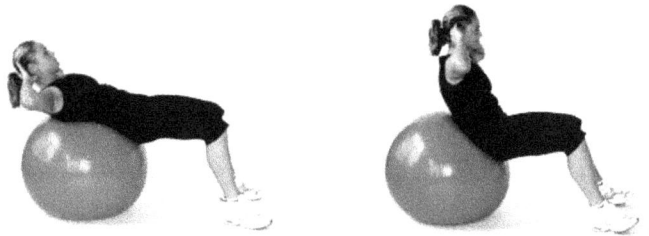

**SIT UP
SUPINE ON THE BALL**

Primary muscles:
Rectus abdominis,
obliques externus and
internus,
transversus abdominis

**CRUNCH ROLL
WITH THE BALL
SUPINE ON THE FLOOR**

Primary muscles:
Rectus abdominis,
obliques externus and internus

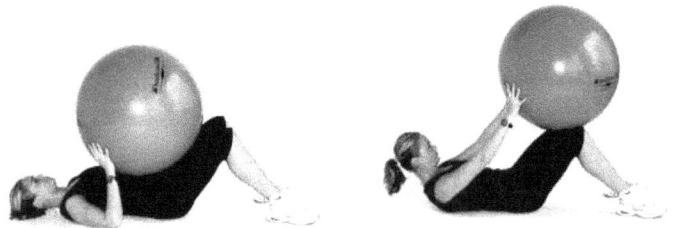

**AB CURL AND
LEG EXTENSION WITH BALL
SUPINE ON THE FLOOR**

Primary muscles:
Rectus abdominis, obliques
externus and internus,
quadriceps

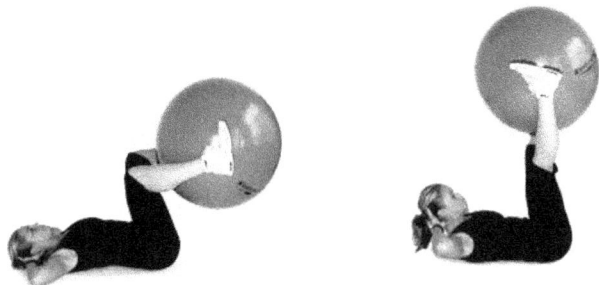

Supine on the ball. Feet on the floor, shoulder-width or wider apart. Hands forward, on the chest, by the head or overhead. Contract the abdominals and curl up the torso. Lower with control.	If needed roll to a semi-supine position, with the lower back and the shoulder blades resting on the ball. The exercise changes, becomes easier, and the head does not move so far backwards. Neck in neutral position. Contract the pelvic floor muscles along with the abs.	Different arm/body/leg position. Arms down in front of the body or overhead (easy to hard). Feet wide apart or together, or on one leg (easy to difficult). Or: The feet up against a wall.
Supine on the ball. Feet on the floor, shoulder-width or wider apart. Hands forward, on the chest, by the head or overhead. Contract the abdominals and then the hip flexors, to perform a sit up. Lower.	If needed roll to a semi-supine position, with the lower back and the shoulder blades resting on the ball. The exercise changes, becomes easier, and the head does not move so far backwards. Neck in neutral position. Contract the pelvic floor muscles along with the abs.	Different arm/body/leg position. Arms down in front of the body or overhead (easy to hard). Feet wide apart or together, or on one leg (easy to difficult).
Supine on the floor. Legs bent and feet on the floor. Stability ball on the stomach, hands on the ball. Contract the abdominals to curl up the torso, so the ball rolls upwards on the thighs. Lower.	Neck in neutral position. Contract the pelvic floor muscles along with the abs. Keep the contraction, do not relax, when the shoulder blades touch the floor.	Different arm/body/leg position.
Supine on the floor. Hips bent, thighs vertical. Knees bent 90 degrees. The stability ball is held between the lower legs. Contract the abs and curl up, at the same time extend the knees, lower legs to vertical. Lower the torso and bend the legs. Return.	Neck in neutral position. Contract the pelvic floor muscles along with the abs. Keep the contraction, do not relax, when the shoulder blades touch the floor.	Different arm position. **OBLIQUE CURL AND LEG EXTENSION** Same exercise, but twist to the side using the obliques. Do one set and change side. Or alternate from side to side.

**V-SIT, BENT LEGS
WITH THE BALL
SITTING ON THE FLOOR**

Primary muscles:
Rectus abdominis, obliques,
iliopsoas, rectus femoris,
transversus abd., multifidii

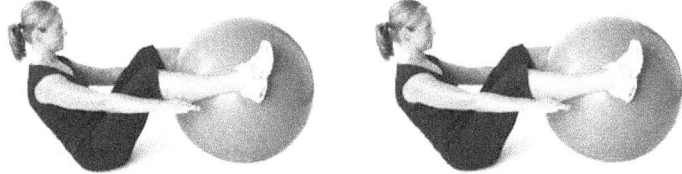

**V-SIT, STRAIGHT LEGS
WITH THE BALL
SITTING ON THE FLOOR**

Primary muscles:
Rectus abdominis, obliques,
iliopsoas, quads, transversus
abdominis, multifidii

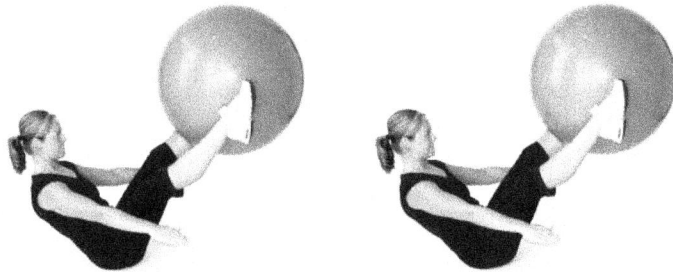

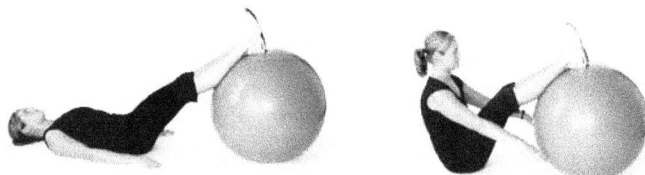

**V-SIT WITH LEGPRESS
WITH THE BALL
SITTING ON THE FLOOR**

Primary muscles: Rectus
abdominis, obliques, quads,
iliopsoas, transversus
abdominis, multifidii

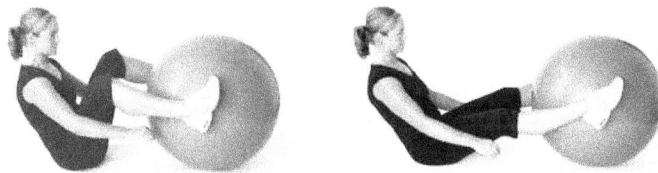

**CURL UP AND SIT UP
FEET ON THE BALL
SUPINE ON THE FLOOR**

Primary muscles:
Rectus abdominis, obliques,
iliopsoas, quads, transversus
abdominis, multifidii

Sitting in balance on the floor. Legs bent and lifted off the floor. The ball is held between the legs and lifted off the floor. Contract the core muscles. The arms are down or forward by the side of the legs. Hold the position.	Isometric exercise. For balance and stabiliztion. Contract the core muscles to stabilize. Contract the pelvic floor muscles. Remember to keep breathing.	Different arm/body/leg position. Rock the body back and forth or from side to side.
Sitting in balance on the floor. Legs straight, in a V-position. The ball is between the legs. Contract the core muscles. The arms are down or forward by the side of the legs. Hold the position.	For intermediate exercisers. Requires some hamstring flexibility. For balance and stabilization. Contract the core muscles to stabilize. Contract the pelvic floor muscles. Remember to keep breathing.	Different arm/body/leg position.
Sitting in balance on the floor. Legs straight and lifted with a stability ball between the feet. The ball is on the floor. Bend the legs and pull the ball towards the body. Contract the core muscles to stabilize and keep the torso upright throughout the exercise. Return.	For balance and stabilization and isometric ab work. Contract the core muscles to stabilize. Contract the pelvic floor muscles. Keep breathing.	Different arm/body/leg position.
Supine on the floor. Feet on the stability ball. Legs straight. Arms on the floor. Contract the ab muscles and hip flexors and lift the torso to upright position. Lower the torso again, rolling down, vertebrae by vertebrae.	For advanced exercisers. Requires some hamstring flexibility. Contract the core muscles to stabilize. Contract the pelvic floor muscles. Avoid letting the hip flexors do all the work (they do the sit up part). Initiate with a curl up.	Different arm position. Legs bent or straight.

**BODY EXTENSION
AND CRUNCH
PRONE ON THE BALL**

Primary muscles:
Gluteus maximus, hamstrings,
rectus abdominis, obliques,
transversus abd., multifidii

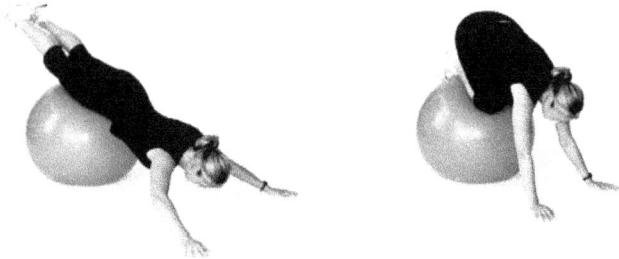

**PELVIC TILT
PLANK POSITION
LOWER LEGS ON THE BALL**

Primary muscles:
Rectus abdominis, obliques,
deltoids, quadriceps,
transversus abd., multifidii

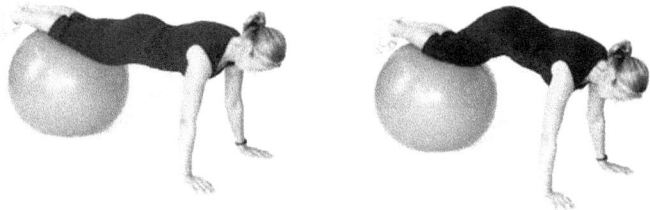

**A-FRAME
PLANK POSITION
FEET ON THE BALL**

Primary muscles:
Rectus abdominis, obliques,
quadriceps, iliopsoas,
transversus abd., multifidii

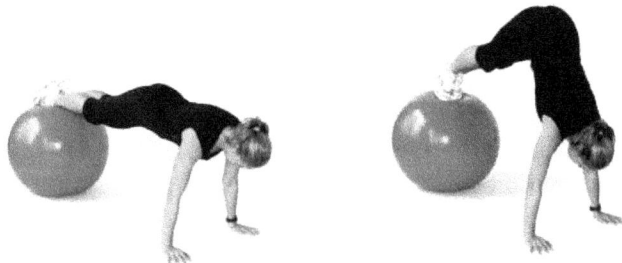

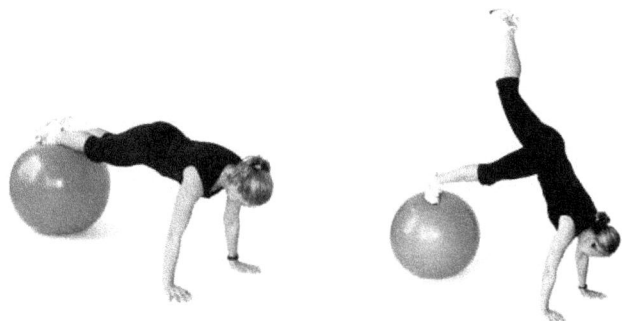

**A-FRAME ON ONE LEG
PLANK POSITION
ONE LEG ON THE BALL**

Primary muscles:
Rectus abdominis, obliques,
quadriceps, iliopsoas,
transversus abd., multifidii

Plank position. Hands on the floor. Lower legs on the ball. Push backwards, so the torso and straight arms get close to the floor, while the legs lift into hip extension. Pull forward into plank position and then pull in the knees to a crunch on the ball.	Total body movement with alternating extension and flexion. Contract the core muscles to stabilize. Keep the neck in neutral position.	Different leg position.
Plank position. Hands on the floor. Lower legs pressed into the ball, the knees are off the ball. Ab muscles contract to perform a pelvic tilt and small curl. Return.	For intermediate exercisers. Contract the core muscles. Watch the wrists.	Different arm/leg position.
Plank position. Lower legs or toes on the ball. Hands on the floor. Contract the abdominals and hip flexors and pull the legs and the ball closer to the hands and the torso. The body forms an A-position. Legs are straight if possible. Return with control.	For advanced exercisers. Requires some hamstring flexibility. Contract the core muscles to stabilize. Keep the neck in neutral position. Watch the wrists.	Different arm position.
Plank position with one lower leg on the ball. Other leg free, lifted slightly above the ball. Contract the abdominals and the hip flexors and pull the leg and the ball closer to the hands and the torso. The body forms an A-position. Legs are straight if possible. Return with control.	For very advanced exercisers. Requires some hamstring flexibility. Contract the core muscles to stabilize. Keep the neck in neutral position. Watch the wrists.	Different arm position. The free leg can be right above the stability ball or be lifted, extended, high in the air into a vertical split position.

**TORSO ROTATION
SITTING ON THE BALL**

Primary muscles:
Obliques externus and
internus,
transversus abdominis,
rotators

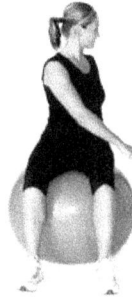

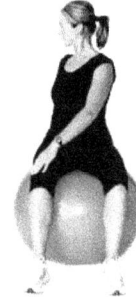

**TORSO ROTATION
SITTING ON THE BALL
WITH ONE LEG LIFTED**

Primary muscles:
Obliques, transversus
abdominis, multifidii, rotators,
quadriceps

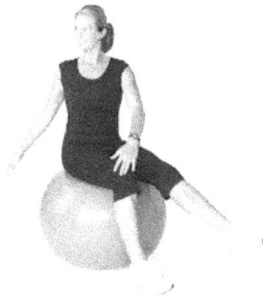

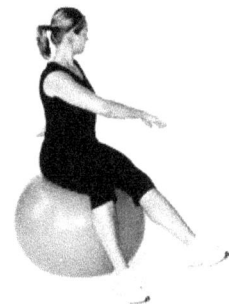

**TORSO ROTATION
SITTING, UNSUPPORTED,
ON THE BALL**

Primary muscles:
Obliques externus and
internus, transversus
abdominis, multifidii, rotators

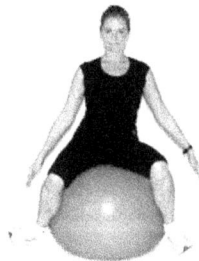

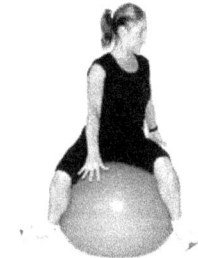

**SIDE/HIP PRESS
KNEELING BY THE BALL**

Primary muscles:
Obliques externus and
internus, quadriceps,
gluteus maximus

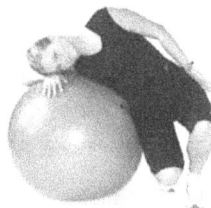

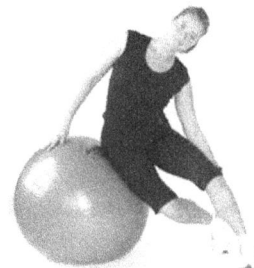

Sitting on the ball. Both feet on the floor. Arms by the side, to the side or folded in front of the chest. Contract the obliques and rotate the torso to the side. Return to center and repeat other side.	Contract the core muscles to stabilize. Torso is erect. Rotate with control.	Different arm/leg position. With the heels or the toes raised.
Sitting on the ball. One foot on the floor, the other leg straight, or bent, and lifted off the floor. Arms to the side or folded in front of the chest. Contract the obliques and rotate the torso to the side. Return to neutral and repeat other side.	Contract the core muscles to stabilize. One leg is kept lifted during rotation right and left. After a set change leg. Torso is erect. Rotate with control.	Different arm/leg position.
Sitting on the ball. Both feet are lifted off the floor. Arms by the side, to side or folded in front of the chest. Contract the obliques and rotate the torso to the side. Return to neutral and repeat other side.	Contract the core muscles to stabilize. Torso is erect. Rotate with control.	Different arm/leg position.
Kneeling by the side of the ball. Lean the torso sideways across the ball. Contract the obliques to bend the torso sideways away from the ball and extend the legs and push the hip sideways into the ball. Return to the starting position. Repeat.	Contract the core muscles to stabilize. Focus on the obliques on the side away from the ball. Contract the thighs to protect the knees. Keep the feet firmly on the ground and watch that the ball does not slip away.	Different arm/leg position.

**OBLIQUE CURL ROLL
WITH THE BALL
SUPINE ON THE FLOOR**

Primary muscles:
Rectus abdominis,
obliques externus and internus

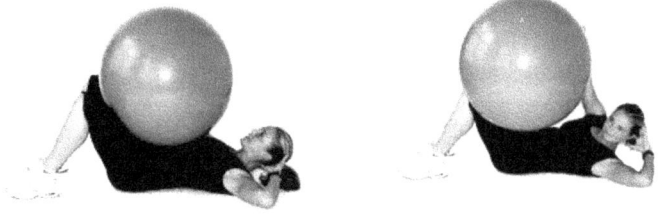

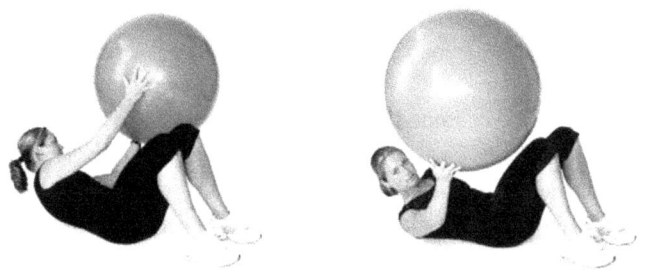

**OBLIQUE CURL
BALL IN HANDS
SUPINE ON THE FLOOR**

Primary muscles:
Rectus abdominis,
obliques externus and internus

**CURL DOWN (ROLL DOWN)
AND ROTATION WITH BALL
SITTING ON THE FLOOR**

Primary muscles:
Obliques externus and
internus, transversus
abdominis, multifidii

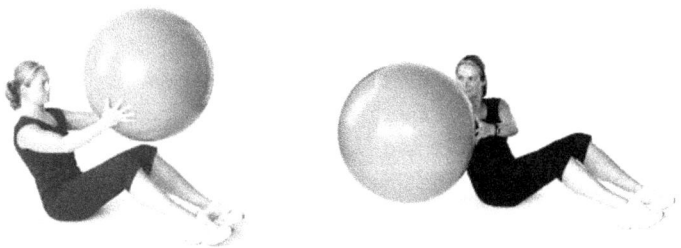

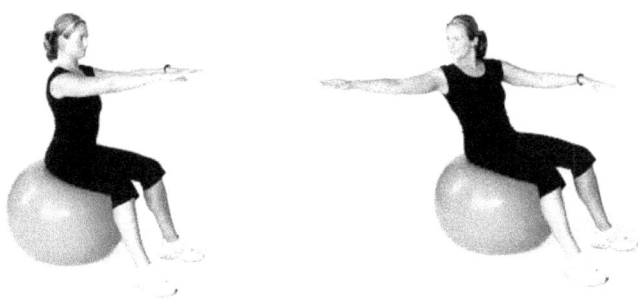

**CURL DOWN (ROLL DOWN)
WITH TORSO ROTATION
SITTING ON THE BALL**

Primary muscles:
Obliques externus and
internus, transversus
abdominis, multifidii

Supine on the floor. Legs bent and feet on the floor. One hand behind the head with upper arm on the floor. The other hand holds the ball. Curl up and rotate the torso diagonally together with the ball. Lower. Repeat. After a set repeat to the other side.	Contract the core muscles to stabilize. Avoid pulling the head with the hands. Keep the neck in neutral position. Contract the pelvic floor muscles along with the abs.	Different arm/leg position.
Supine on the floor. Legs bent and feet on the floor. The hands hold a stability ball. Contract the obliques and lift and twist to one side together with the ball. Lower. Repeat. After a set repeat to the other side.	Contract the core muscles to stabilize. Neck in neutral position. Contract the pelvic floor muscles along with the abs.	Different arm/leg position. The arms may be forward, vertical or by the head.
Sitting on the floor. Legs bent. The stability ball is in the hands. Roll the torso down, vertebrae by vertebrae. Midway in the movement rotate the torso to the side. Rotate back to neutral. Roll up. Roll down and repeat to the opposite side. (Or stay down and rotate left and right).	Contract the core muscles to stabilize. Neck in neutral position. Contract the pelvic floor muscles along with the abs.	Different arm/leg position. The stability ball may be held close to the body or away from from the body.
Sitting on the ball. The arms straight forward in front of the chest. Roll the torso down, vertebrae by vertebrae. Halfway down rotate the torso to the side. Rotate back to neutral. Roll up. Roll down and repeat to the opposite side. (Or stay down and rotate left and right).	Contract the core muscles to stabilize. Neck in neutral position. Contract the pelvic floor muscles along with the abs.	Different arm/leg position.

**OBLIQUE CURL
SUPINE ON THE BALL**

Primary muscles:
Rectus abdominis,
obliques externus and
internus, transversus
abdominis, multifidii

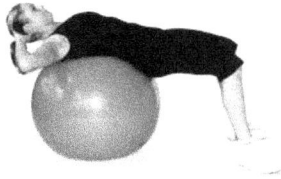

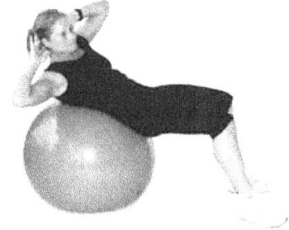

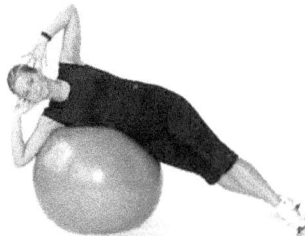

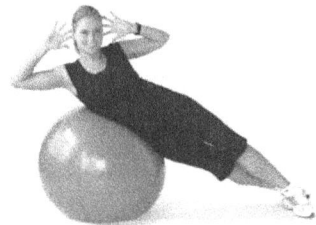

**OBLIQUE CURL
WITH OPPOSITE LEG LIFT
SUPINE ON THE BALL**

Primary muscles:
Rectus abdominis, obliques,
transversus abdominis,
multifidii

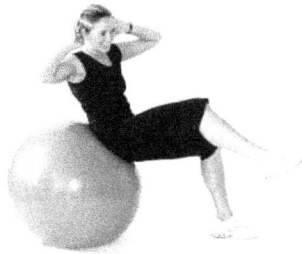

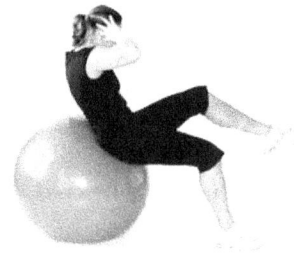

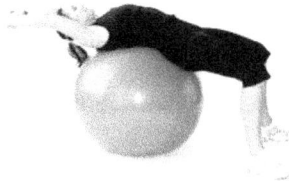

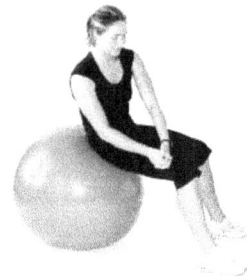

**OBLIQUE CURL WITH
ARM PULL (WOOD CHOP)
SUPINE ON THE BALL**

Primary muscles:
Rectus abdominis, obliques,
transversus abdominis,
multifidii

**TORSO SIDE FLEXION
SIDELYING ON THE BALL**

Primary muscles:
Obliques externus and
internus, transversus
abdominis, multifidi

Supine on the ball. Feet on the floor. Hands forward, by the chest, by the head or overhead. Contract the obliques and curl up and rotate. Move the shoulder diagonally towards the opposite hip. Lower. Repeat or repeat to the opposite side.	If needed use a semi-supine position, with the lower back and the shoulder blades resting on the ball. The exercise changes, becomes easier, and the head does not move so far backwards. Contract the core muscles. Contract the pelvic floor muscles along with the abs.	Different arm/body/leg position. Arms down in front of the body or overhead (easy or hard). The arms are passive or active. Feet wide apart or together, or on one leg (easy to difficult).
Supine on the ball. The feet on the floor. Hands by the chest or by the head. Contract the obliques and curl up and rotate. At the same time lift the leg you are twisting toward. Lower. Repeat or repeat to the opposite side.	Contract the core muscles to stabilize. Contract the pelvic floor muscles along with the abs. At first lift only the heel off the floor, then the foot and finally the leg (knee).	Different arm position. The arms down in front of the body or overhead (easier or harder). The arms are passive or active. Feet wide apart or together, or on one leg (easy to difficult).
Supine on the ball. Feet on the floor. Straight arms overhead. Curl up the torso and twist diagonally to one side. The arms move diagonally across the body to the side of the leg. Lower the torso and arms back down. Repeat or repeat to the opposite side.	If needed use a semi-supine position, with the lower back and the shoulder blades resting on the ball. The exercise changes, becomes easier, and the head does not move so far backwards. Contract the pelvic floor muscles along with the abs.	Different leg position. With or without a dumbbell in the hands.
Sidelying. Feet are staggered on the floor. Hands by the head or on the chest. Contract the obliques to sidebend in the frontal plane. Lower backwards to the starting position.	Contract the core muscles. Keep the body in the frontal plane and lift straight to the side. Avoid crunching or arching the back. The feet may slip on the floor, to avoid this use a yoga mat. Or anchor them by a wall(bar), but then you take away most of the balance work.	Different arm/leg position. When the feet are on the floor, the focus is on balance work and the obliques. When the feet are anchored by a wall or wall bar, the focus is on the quadratus lumborum and less balance work.

**TORSO TWIST
FROM SUPINE TO TWISTED
BRIDGE ON THE BALL**

Primary muscles:
Obliques externus and
internus, transversus
abdominis, multifidii

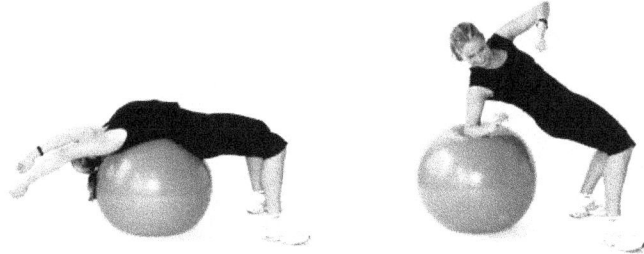

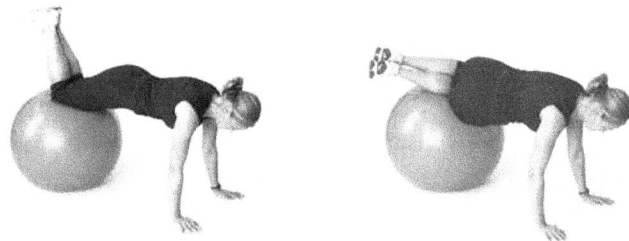

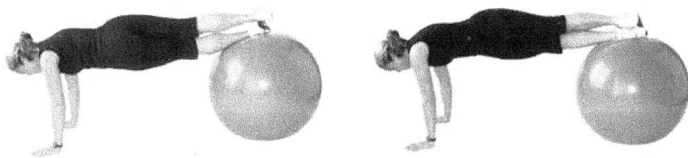

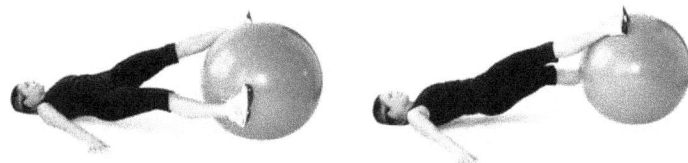

**HIP TWIST WITH BALL
PLANK, BENT LEGS,
THIGHS ON THE BALL**

Primary muscles:
Obliques externus and
internus, transversus
abdominis, multifidii

**HIP TWIST WITH BALL
PLANK POSITION
LOWER LEGS ON THE BALL**

Primary muscles:
Obliques externus and
internus, transversus
abdominis, multifidii

**HIP TWIST
LEGS HOLD THE BALL
SUPINE ON THE FLOOR**

Primary muscles:
Obliques externus and
internus, transversus
abdominis, multifidii

Supine on the ball. Feet on the floor. Arms straight back behind the head. Contract the abs and the biceps to lift the body up into a sideplank position on one forearm. Lower back down and repeat to the other side.	For intermediate exercisers. Contract the core muscles to stabilize. Neck in neutral position.	Different arm position.
Plank position. Thighs on the ball, knees bent 90 degrees, legs press into the ball. Hands on the floor. Contract the obliques to rotate the hips and legs to one side, Repeat to the other side.	Contract the core muscles to stabilize. Neck in neutral position. Watch the wrists. The wrists should be strengthened gradually with few repetitions initially, short lever and more rests between sets.	Different arm/leg position.
Plank position. Hands on the floor. Feet on top of the ball. Keep legs together and the body on a long straight line, then it is much easier to keep the balance. Contract the obliques to rotate the hips and legs to the side. Repeat to the other side.	Contract the core muscles to stabilize. Neck in neutral position. Watch the wrists. The wrists should be strengthened gradually with few repetitions initially, short lever and rests between sets.	Different arm position.
Supine on the floor. Legs straight, feet on each side of the ball. Arms on the floor. Contract the obliques, so the body, legs and ball rotate to the side. Repeat to the other side.	Contract the core muscles to stabilize. Neck in neutral position.	Different arm/leg position.

**SCISSORS WITH THE BALL
SUPINE ON THE FLOOR**

Primary muscles:
Transversus abdominis,
multifidii, adductors,
quadriceps, iliopsoas

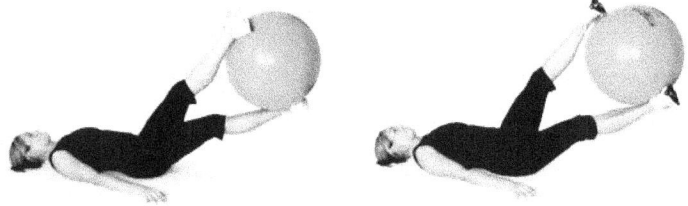

**SCISSORS WITH THE BALL
SIDELYING ON THE FLOOR**

Primary muscles:
Obliques externus and
internus,
transversus abdominis,
multifidii, adductors

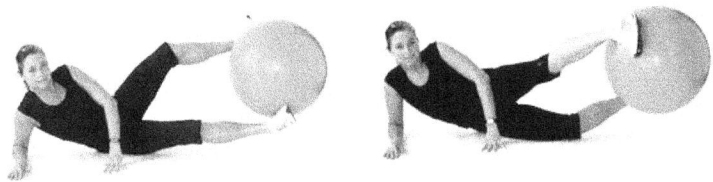

**SCISSORS (PENDULUM)
WITH ROTATION
SUPINE ON THE FLOOR**

Primary muscles:
Hip muscles,
transversus abdominis,
multifidii

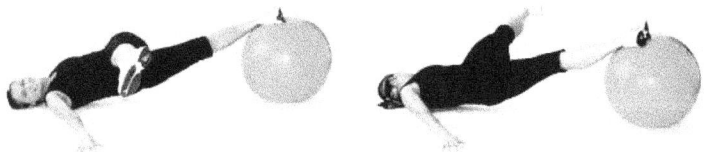

**SCISSORS
WITH ROTATION
PLANK POSITION**

Primary muscles:
Hip muscles,
transversus abdominis,
multifidii, deltoids

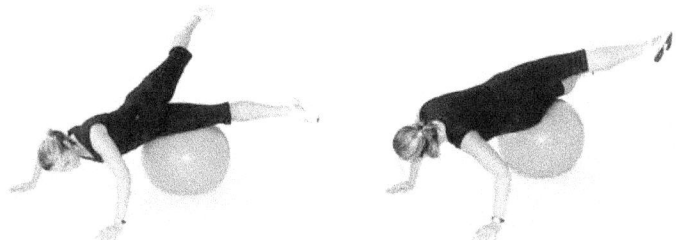

Supine on the floor. Arms on the floor. The lower legs hold and squeeze the ball. The legs are lifted off the floor. Legs scissor, cross over and under each other, to rotate the stability ball. Core muscles contract to keep the body stable.	For advanced exercisers. Some core strength is needed to keep the lower back from arching, when straight legs are lifted – a heavy load. A slow to moderate tempo is recommended. Contract the core muscles to stabilize.	Different arm position.
Sidelying on the floor. The lower legs hold and squeeze the ball, legs are lifted off the floor. Arms on the floor to stabilize the body. Legs scissor, cross over and under each other, to rotate the stability ball. Core muscles contract to keep the body stable.	For intermediate exercisers. Some core strength is needed to keep the body stable and avoid rotating the spine excessively. A slow to moderate tempo is recommended. Contract the core to stabilize.	Different arm/leg position.
Bridge. Upper back on the floor. One lower leg on the ball. Other leg is lifted above the ball. The top lifted leg crosses over the leg on the ball and at the same time the hip rotates. The lower leg moves backward with the ball, a scissor move. Return and repeat or repeat other side.	For intermediate exercisers. The arms and the upper back stay on the floor. Original Klein-Vogelbach exercise, that mobilizes and strengthens the hip muscles.	Different arm position.
Prone on the ball. Thighs on the ball, legs together. Hands wide apart on the floor. Rotate the head towards one hand, rotate the pelvis to the same side. The legs open in a sidelying scissor movement forward/backward. The head turns towards the opposite hand, repeat opposite side.	For intermediate exercisers. Hands are firmly on the floor. Keep the torso stable. The head stays in the same position, level, above the floor. Original Klein-Vogelbach exercise, that mobilizes and strengthens the muscles in the torso and the hips.	Different arm/leg position.

TORSO ROTATION
BRIDGE POSITION

Primary muscles:
Obliques externus and
internus, gluteus maximus,
hamstrings, transversus
abdominis, multifidii

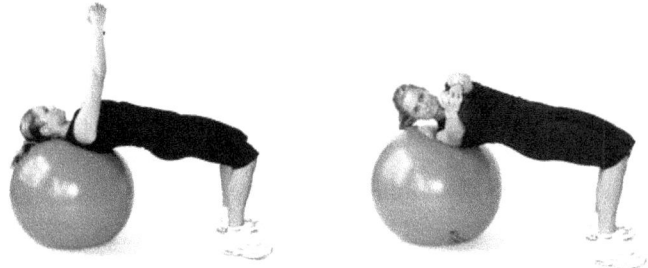

RUSSIAN TWIST
WITH STABILITY BALL
SUPINE ON THE FLOOR

Primary muscles:
Rectus abdominis, obliques
externus and internus,
transversus abdominis

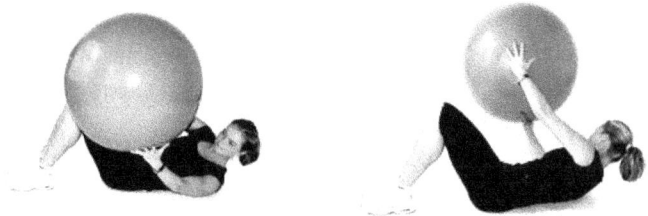

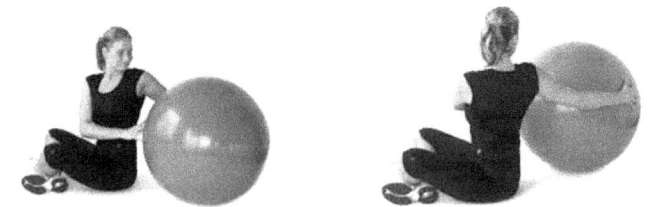

TORSO ROTATION
WITH STABILITY BALL
SITTING ON THE FLOOR

Primary muscles:
Obliques externus and
internus,
transversus abdominis

OBLIQUE CURL
(BALL CRUNCH) WITH KICK
SUPINE ON THE BALL

Primary muscles:
Rectus abdominis, obliques,
transversus abdominis,
multifidii, iliopsoas, quadriceps

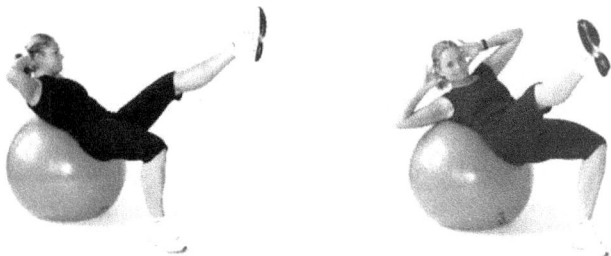

Bridge position. Shoulder blades on the ball. Legs bent and feet on the floor. The arms are vertical with the hands together. Obliques contract to rotate the torso and arms to one side. Return and repeat opposite.	Contract the core muscles to stabilize. The torso and shoulder press into the stability ball to create resistance.	Different body/leg position. With a dumbbell or medicine ball in the hands.
Supine on the floor. The hips and legs are bent. Feet on the floor. Hold the stability ball in the hands, arms are slightly bent. Lift the torso and rotate right to left with the stability ball.	For advanced exercisers. A slow to moderate tempo is recommended. The rectus abdominis should be contracted throughout the exercise to protect the back.	Different leg position. With a dumbbell or medicine ball In the hands.
Sitting on the floor. The ball is in the hands. Rotate the torso as far back as possible. Put the ball on the floor and quickly rotate to the other side and pick up the the ball and rotate and put it down again. Repeat. After a set, change and rotate the opposite way.	Contract the core muscles to stabilize. Keep the torso erect. Rotate with control.	Different leg position. **BACK TO BACK ROTATION WITH A PARTNER** Standing back to back with a partner. You rotate and pass the ball to the partner.
Supine. One foot on the floor. Other leg straight (or bent), heel resting lightly on the floor. One hand behind the head, other hand around the ball (or behind the head). Curl up and rotate the torso towards the opposite leg, which lifts at the same time. Lower. Repeat. After a set repeat opposite.	Contract the core muscles to stabilize. Contract the pelvic floor muscles along with the abs.	Different arm position.

**FLATTEN BACK
WITH BALL BETWEEN LEGS
SUPINE ON THE FLOOR**

Primary muscles:
Quadriceps, iliopsoas,
transversus abdominis,
multifidii

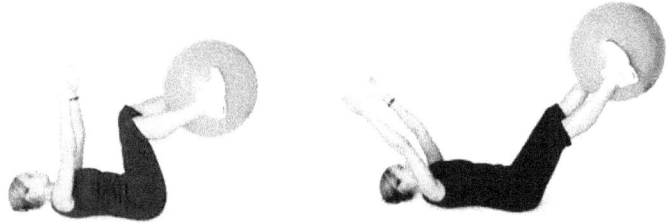

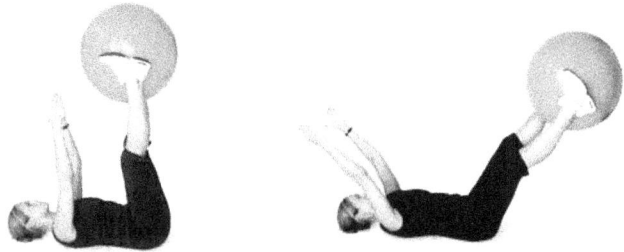

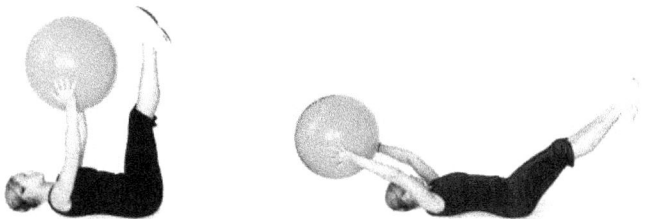

**ARM AND LEG LIFT
WITH BALL BETWEEN LEGS
SUPINE ON THE FLOOR**

Primary muscles:
Quadriceps, iliopsoas
transversus abdominis,
multifidii

**ARM AND LEG LIFT
WITH BALL IN THE HANDS
SUPINE ON THE FLOOR**

Primary muscles:
Quadriceps, iliopsoas,
transversus abdominis,
multifidii

**PLANK TO PIKE POSITION,
PLANK POSITION
FOREARMS ON THE BALL**

Primary muscles:
Rectus abdominis, iliopsoas,
obliques, transversus
abdominis, multifidii

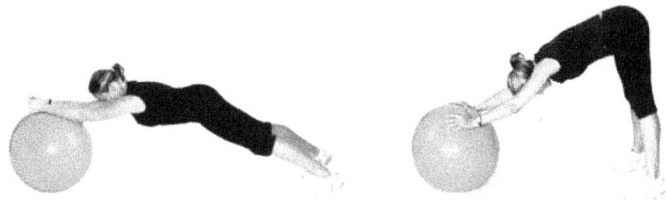

Supine. The arms are vertical. Hips and knees are flexed 90 degrees, tabletop position. The ball is held by the feet. Lower the arms behind the head, legs towards the floor. Contract the abs and core to keep the lower back in neutral position. Return the arms and thighs to vertical position.	For intermediate exercisers. A slow to moderate tempo is recommended. Contract the core and abs throught the exercise to keep the lower back in neutral position. Contract the pelvic floor.	Different arm/leg position. With a dumbbell or medicine ball in the hands.
Supine. Legs and arms are vertical. The stability ball is held by the feet. Lower the arms behind the head, legs towards the floor. Contract the abs and core to keep the lower back in neutral position. Return the arms and legs to vertical position.	For advanced exercisers. A slow to moderate tempo is recommended. Contract the core and abs throught the exercise to keep the lower back in neutral position. Contract the pelvic floor.	Different arm/leg position.
Supine. Legs and arms are vertical. The stability ball is held by the hands. Lower the arms behind the head, legs towards the floor. Contract abs and core to keep the lower back in neutral position. Return to vertical position.	For advanced exercisers. A slow to moderate tempo is recommended. Contract the core and abs throught the exercise to keep the lower back in neutral position. Contract the pelvic floor.	Different arm/leg position.
Plank position. Forearms on the ball. Contract the abs to pull the torso closer to the legs. Return with control.	For very advanced exercisers. Hard on the shoulders. Contract the core muscles to stabilize. Neck in neutral position.	Different arm/leg position.

KNEE TUCK WITH TWIST
PLANK POSITION
LEGS ON THE BALL

Primary muscles:
Rectus abdominis, obliques,
transversus abdominis,
multifidii, iliopsoas, quadriceps

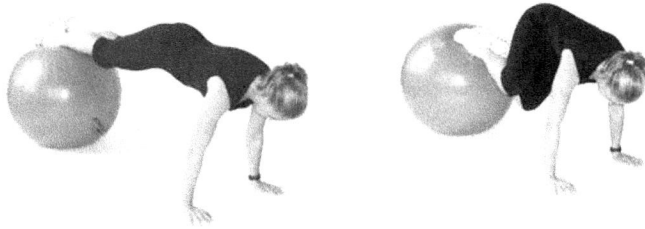

SIDELEAN ISOMETRIC
(FRONTAL PLANE LEAN)
SIDELYING ON THE BALL

Primary muscles:
Obliques, quadratus
lumborum, transversus
abdominis, multifidii

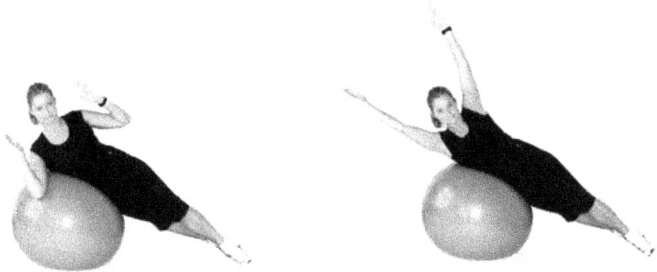

BRIDGE, DYNAMIC
BRIDGE POSITION

Primary muscles:
Gluteus maximus, hamstrings,
erector spinae,
transversus abdominis,
multifidii

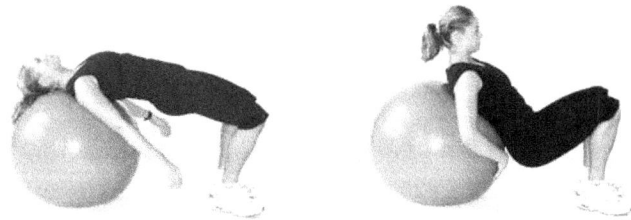

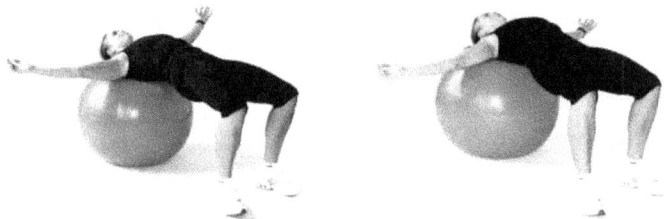

BRIDGE T-POSITION
LATERAL ROLL
BRIDGE POSITION

Primary muscles:
Gluteus maximus, hamstrings,
erector spinae, transversus
abdominis, multifidii

Plank position. Hands on the floor. Feet or lower legs on the ball. Contract the abs and pull the knees towards the torso and diagonally to the side. In the last part of the movement do a pelvic tilt. Return. Press the legs into the ball for resistance. Repeat to the other side.	Contract the core muscles to stabilize. In the last part of the movement contract the lower part of the abs, do a pelvic tilt. Watch the wrists. The wrists should be strengthened gradually.	Different arm position. With both legs or one leg (for very advanced exercisers).
Sidelying on the ball. The feet are staggered on the floor. Hold the body in a diagonal position. You can do various arm movements in this position.	Contract the core muscles to stabilize. Keep breathing. The feet may slip on the floor, to avoid this use a yoga mat. Or anchor them by a wall(bar), but then you take away most of the balance work.	Different arm/leg position.
Bridge position. Arms relaxed. Feet on the floor. Shins in vertical position throughout the exercise. Keep the buttocks contracted and lift and lower the hips in a dynamic bridge motion. The upper back and the head should stay on the ball (not lifted as in the right photo).	Contract the core muscles to stabilize. Contract the buttocks in the top position. For more glute work, keep the position for 2-3 seconds.	Different arm/leg position. **BRIDGE WITH ONE LEG** Supine. Shoulder blades on top of the ball. The body in bridge position, one foot on the floor, the knee bent 90 degrees. Other leg extended. Lower the buttocks. Keep the free leg straight and parallel to the floor.
Bridge position. Upper back on top of the ball. Feet on the floor hip-width apart. Arms to the side in horizontal plane, T-position. Keep the body level and roll the torso slightly sideways on the ball, return and repeat to the opposite side.	Contract the core muscles to stabilize. Keep the hips level. Perform a slow movement from side to side.	T-position with or without leg movement; the feet stay on the spot or the feet move, so the legs move to the side along with the ball. Change direction; a few steps to the left and a few steps to the right.

FORWARD BALL ROLL
KNEELING ON THE FLOOR

Primary muscles:
Transversus abdominis,
multifidii, deltoids,
latissimus dorsi

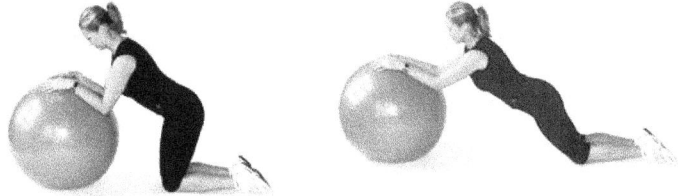

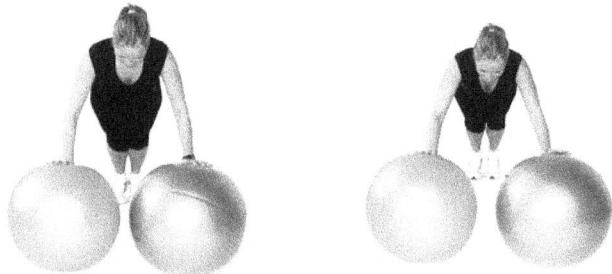

ROLL OUT, TWO BALLS
PLANK POSITION
HANDS ON TWO BALLS

Primary muscles:
Transversus abdominis,
multifidii, deltoids,
latissimus dorsi

ROCK'N'ROLL
SITTING ON THE FLOOR

Primary muscles:
Rectus abdominis, obliques,
erector spinae, transversus
abdominis, multifidii

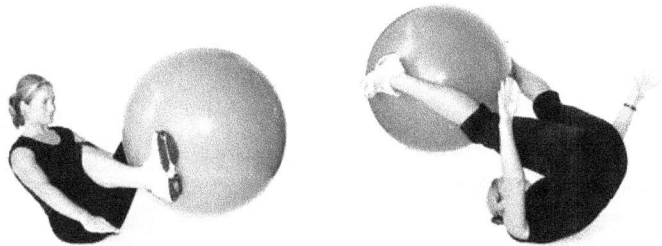

BALL WALK AROUND
(CLOCK WALKS), PLANK,
HANDS ON THE FLOOR

Primary muscles:
Transversus abdominis,
multifidii, rectus abdominis,
deltoids, triceps brachii

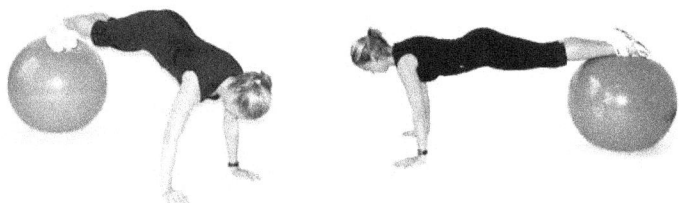

Kneeling behind the ball. Hips flexed approx. 90 degrees. Forearms and hands on the ball. Contract the core and roll forward. Hips and shoulders open up at the same time. The arms roll forward on the ball, so the angle between the arm and torso increases. Move into plank position. Return.	For intermediate exercisers. Contract the core muscles to stabilize. Avoid arching the lower back or piking the buttocks. Can be performed dynamically or isometrically, holding the end position.	On the lower legs or the toes. With two arms or: With one arm (for advanced exercisers). In the end range of motion the stability ball may be rolled from side to side, in figure eights or other patterns.
Plank position. Feet on the floor. One hand on each ball. Contract the core muscles. Roll the stability balls forward with a small, slow, controlled movement. Return with control.	For advanced exercisers. Contract the core muscles to stabilize. The range of motion is limited, approx. 20-30 cm forward and backward (or the hands will roll off the ball).	Different leg position. **ASYMMETRIC ROLL OUT** For very advanced exercisers: Start in push-up position with a hand – or forearm – on each ball. One ball is rolled forward and the other backward.
Sitting in a balance on the floor. Legs bent and lifted off the floor, feet hold the ball. Arms forward by the side of the legs. The body rolls down onto the upper back, legs straighten parallel to the floor. Return. Roll back up to seated position.	For intermediate exercisers. Fun exercise with a stopping action and a hold. Balance and core work. Contract the core muscles to stabilize. Stop when rolling onto the shoulder blades, do not roll onto the cervical vertebrae.	Different range of motion, from a small roll to a big movement all the way into plough position with the legs past the head (for advanced exercisers). Legs can be bent throughout the movement.
Plank position. Feet on the ball. Hands on the floor. Walk with the hands, a full circle around the stability ball. The feet also move, just a little or perform a 'walk' on top of the ball. Repeat the opposite way around.	For advanced exercisers. Contract the core muscles to stabilize. Hips are level. Neck in neutral position. Progression: Start with a ¼ or ½ circle walk. Watch the wrists.	Different leg position.

RAINBOWS
SUPINE ON THE FLOOR
LEGS ON THE BALL

Primary muscles:
Obliques externus and
internus, transversus
abdominis, multifidii

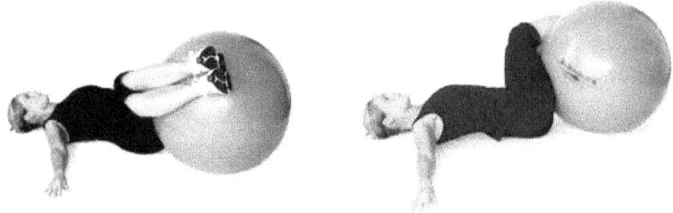

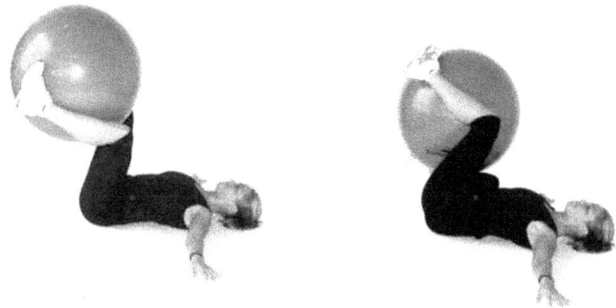

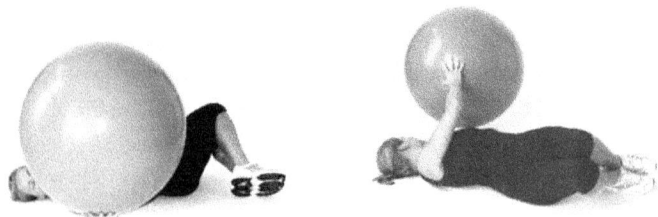

RAINBOWS, BENT LEGS
LEGS HOLDING THE BALL
SUPINE ON THE FLOOR

Primary muscles:
Obliques externus and
internus, transversus
abdominis, multifidii

RAINBOWS,
STRAIGHT LEGS
LEGS HOLDING THE BALL
SUPINE ON THE FLOOR

Primary muscles:
Obliques, transversus
abdominis, multifidii

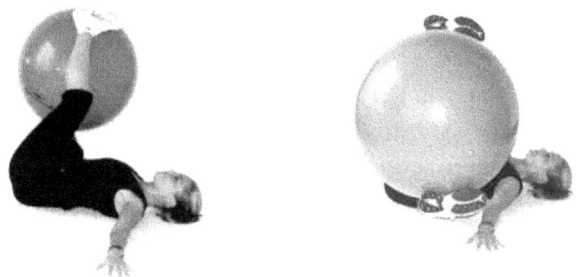

DOUBLE RUSSIAN TWIST
SUPINE ON THE FLOOR

Primary muscles:
Obliques externus and
internus, transversus
abdominis, multifidii

Supine on the floor. Arms to the side to stabilize. Hips and knees bent 90 degrees. Lower legs on the ball, hamstrings against the ball. The lower legs and hamstrings contract to hold the ball. Contract the obliques and lower the legs to one side. Return and repeat other side.	For beginning exercisers and for advanced exercisers as a warm-up. Contract the core to stabilize. Slow to moderate tempo. The torso and the shoulder blades are kept on the floor.	Different arm position. Different range of motion. Start with a small range of motion to prepare the spine for the exercise.
Supine on the floor. Arms to the side to stabilize. Hips and knees bent 90 degrees, tabletop position. Hold the ball between the feet or lower legs. Contract the obliques and lower the legs to one side. Return and repeat to the other side.	For intermediate exercisers. Contract the core muscles to stabilize. A slow tempo is recommended. The arms and the shoulder blades are kept on the floor.	Different arm position. Different range of motion. Start with a small range of motion to prepare the spine for the exercise. Use a medicine ball for more resistance.
Supine on the floor. Arms to the side to stabilize. Legs vertical. 90 degrees of hip flexion, knees straight. The ball is held between the feet and lower legs. Contract the obliques and lower the legs to one side. Return and repeat to the other side.	For advanced exercisers. Contract the core muscles to stabilize. A slow to moderate tempo is recommended. The arms and the shoulder blades are kept on the floor.	Different arm position. Different range of motion. Start with a small range of motion to prepare the spine for the exercise. Use a medicine ball for more resistance.
Supine on the floor. Legs bent with the feet on the floor. The hands hold a ball over the torso. Contract the obliques and lower the bent legs to one side and the arms and the ball to the opposite side. Return and repeat to the opposite side.	Contract the core muscles to stabilize. Keep contracting the obliques to protect the spine. Do not let go in the end ranges of motion. A slow to moderate tempo is recommended.	Different arm position. Use a medicine ball for more resistance. Start with a small range of motion to prepare the spine for the exercise.

**OBLIQUE CURL
WITH BALL PULL
SUPINE ON THE FLOOR**

Primary muscles:
Obliques, rectus abdominis,
hamstrings, gluteus maximus,
transversus abd., multifidii

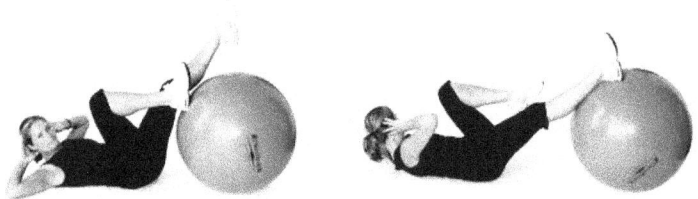

**V-SIT WITH TWIST
SITTING ON THE FLOOR**

Primary muscles:
Obliques externus and
internus, rectus abdominis,
transversus abdominis,
multifidii

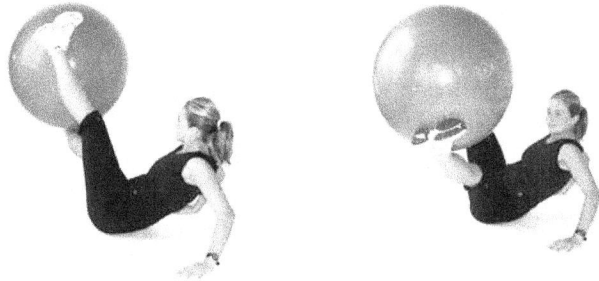

**CURL AND BRIDGE COMBO
SUPINE ON THE FLOOR**

Primary muscles:
Rectus abdominis, obliques
externus and internus,
transversus abd., multifidii
gluteus maximus, hamstrings

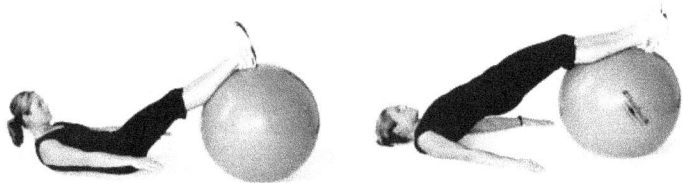

**WIND SCREEN WIPERS
SUPINE ON THE FLOOR**

Primary muscles:
Rectus abdominis, obliques,
iliopsoas, rectus femoris,
transversus abdominis,
multifidii

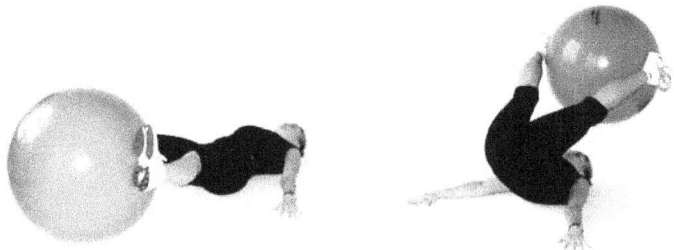

Supine on the floor. Hands by the head. One leg bent, foot on top of the ball. Other leg straight and lifted off the ball/ floor. Bend the free leg, pull it towards the torso and curl towards the knee. At the same time straighten other leg, push ball away from torso. Repeat. After a set repeat other side.	Contract the core muscles to stabilize. A slow speed is recommended in the beginning. Neck in neutral position. Avoid pulling on the head and neck.	Different arm position.
Sitting on the floor. Body in a V-position. Hands on the floor behind the body or at the side. The feet hold the ball. Contract the abdominals and twist the legs from side to side (like Rainbows).	For advanced exercisers. Contract the core muscles to stabilize.	Different arm position. **LEG SWING OVER THE BALL** Sitting in a V-sit position. The ball is on the floor. Lift the legs in a semi-circle from side to side over the stability ball (for advanced exercisers).
Supine on the floor. Legs straight. Lower legs on the ball. Arms on the floor by the side of the body. Contract the ab muscles and curl torso up. Lower the torso. Contract the buttocks and hamstrings and lift into bridge position. Lower. Repeat.	Contract the core muscles to stabilize. Keep the contraction and control throughout exercise; fluent transitions between the two positions. Avoid lifting too high into the bridge position, do not rest on the cervical vertebrae.	Different arm position.
Supine. Legs vertical with a stability ball between the feet. Arms on the floor. Contract the abdominals and the hip flexors and lift the legs over the torso and head. Contract the abs and core muscles and lower the legs down until they are just above the floor. Repeat.	For advanced exercisers. Contract the core muscles to stabilize. Stop when rolling onto the shoulder blades, do not roll onto the cervical vertebrae.	Legs bent or straight.

HIP LIFT
LEGS ON THE BALL
SUPINE ON THE FLOOR

Primary muscles:
Rectus abdominis,
obliques externus and internus

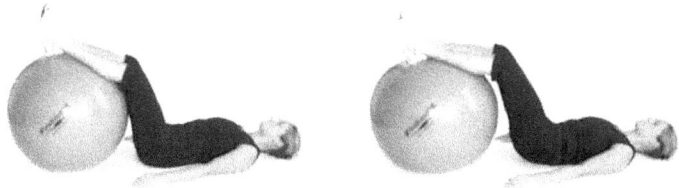

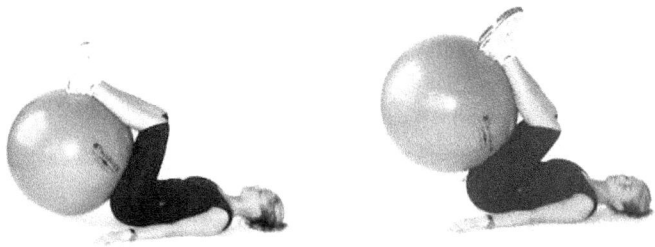

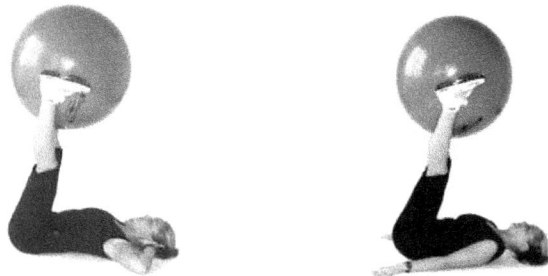

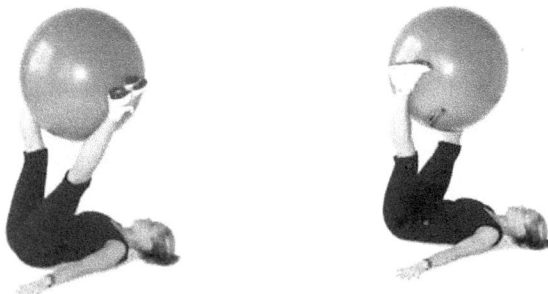

REVERSE CURL
BALL UNDER BENT LEGS
SUPINE ON THE FLOOR

Primary muscles:
Rectus abdominis,
obliques externus and internus

REVERSE CURL WITH BALL
BETWEEN STRAIGHT LEGS
SUPINE ON THE FLOOR

Primary muscles:
Rectus abdominis,
obliques externus and internus

REVERSE CURL WITH TWIST
BALL BETWEEN LEGS
SUPINE ON THE FLOOR

Primary muscles:
Rectus abdominis,
obliques externus and internus

Supine on the floor. Arms on the floor. Lower legs on the ball. Ab muscles, lower part, contract to perform a pelvic tilt. A small isolation movement. Lower.	For beginning to advanced exercisers. Focus is on the lower part of the rectus abdominis. Tilt the pelvis with the ab muscles. Avoid contracting the buttocks, as this changes the exercise and makes it easier.	Different arm/leg position.
Supine on the floor. Legs over the ball. Contract the hamstrings and push the heels into the ball, so it stays in place. Contract the abdominals to perform a reverse ab curl. Lower.	It can be hard to hold the stability ball with the legs, if the stability ball is too big. Use a smaller ball if necessary.	Different arm position.
Supine on the floor. Arms on the floor to stabilize the body. Legs vertical with the ball between the feet. Contract the abdominals to perform a reverse ab curl. Lift the buttocks and legs straight upwards. Lower.	Lift the pelvis with the lower part of the rectus abdominis. Avoid using the hip flexors, do not swing the legs.	Different arm position. Legs straight or bent.
Supine on the floor. Arms on the floor to stabilize the body. Legs vertical with the ball between the feet. Contract the abdominals, lift the pelvis. Keep it lifted and twist the hips from side to side.	Lift the pelvis with the lower part of the rectus abdominis. Avoid using the hip flexors, do not swing the legs.	Different arm position. Legs straight or bent.

**REVERSE CURL WITH CRUNCH
WITH THE BALL
SUPINE ON THE FLOOR**

Primary muscles:
Rectus abdominis, obliques
externus and internus,
transversus abdominis

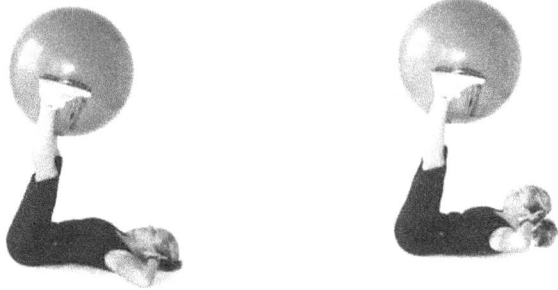

**BRIDGE, DYNAMIC
REVERSE PLANK, HEELS ON
BALL, HANDS ON FLOOR**

Primary muscles:
Gluteus maximus, hamstrings,
erector spinae, deltoids,
transversus abd., multifidii

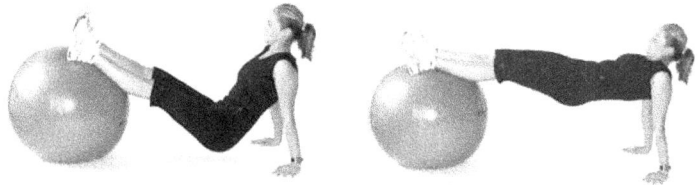

**BRIDGE WITH LOWER LEGS
ON THE BALL
SUPINE ON THE FLOOR**

Primary muscles:
Gluteus maximus, hamstrings,
transversus abdominis,
multifidii

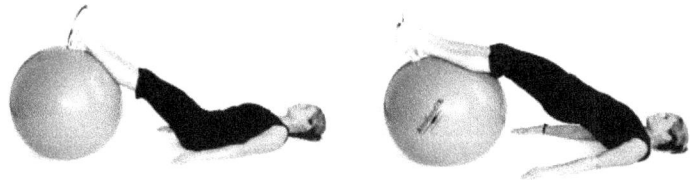

**BRIDGE
WITH HEELS ON THE BALL
SUPINE ON THE FLOOR**

Primary muscles:
Gluteus maximus, hamstrings,
erector spinae, transversus
abdominis, multifidii

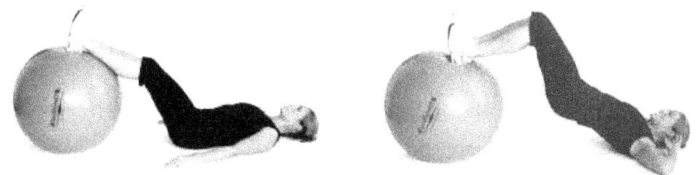

Supine on the floor. Arms forward, by the chest, by the head or overhead. Legs vertical with the ball between the feet. Contract the abdominals and curl up the torso and the pelvis at the same time; a crunch. Lower.	Lift the pelvis with the ab muscles. Avoid using the hip flexors, do not swing the legs. Tip: Focus on contracting the upper and lower part of the abdominals with equal force; 50 % above the navel, 50 % below the navel.	Legs straight or bent.
Sitting on the floor. Hands on the floor behind the body. Heels/lower legs on top of the ball. Legs straight. Contract the buttocks and lift the body into bridge position. Hold or lower and repeat.	For advanced exercisers. Watch the shoulders and wrists. Keep the shoulder girdle stable and the neck 'long', keep the head away from the shoulders. When performing the exercise dynamically, do not touch the buttocks to the floor. Stop right above the floor.	Different arm position. On one or both legs. Same exercise, but when you lower the buttocks, twist the hips back and to one side. Repeat to the other side.
Supine on the floor. Lower legs on the ball. Arms on the floor to stabilize the body. Contract the buttocks and lift the body into bridge position. Keep the shoulders and the upper back on the floor. Hold the position or lower back to the starting position.	Contract the core muscles to stabilize. Keep the hips level. Stop lifting when you reach the shoulder blades, avoid supporting on the cervical vertebrae.	Different arm position. Lift the arms off the floor for increased balance work. On one or both legs.
Supine on the floor. Shoulders and upper back on the floor. Heels on the ball. Contract the buttocks and hamstrings and lift the body into bridge position. Hold the position or lower back to the starting position.	Contract the core muscles to stabilize. Keep the hips level. Stop lifting when you reach the shoulder blades, avoid supporting on the cervical vertebrae.	Different arm position. One on or both legs.

**MARCH ON THE BALL
IN BRIDGE POSITION
SUPINE ON THE FLOOR**

Primary muscles:
Gluteus maximus, hamstrings,
erector spinae, transversus
abdominis, multifidii

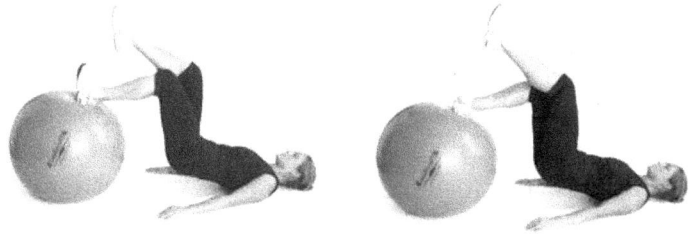

**BRIDGE ON ONE LEG
LOWER LEG ON THE BALL
ONE LEG TO THE SIDE
UPPER BACK ON THE FLOOR**

Primary muscles: Gluteus
maximus, hamstrings, erector
spinae, rotators, t.a., multifidii

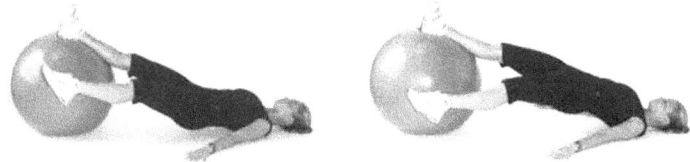

**BRIDGE WITH HIP ROTATION
FEET ON THE BALL
UPPER BACK ON THE FLOOR**

Primary muscles: Obliques,
gluteus maximus, hamstrings,
transversus abdominis,
multifidii

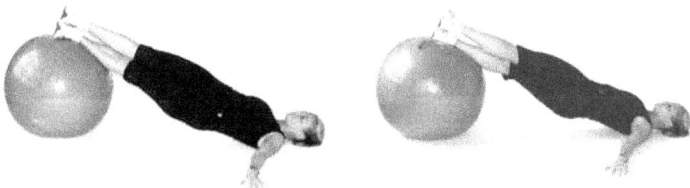

**PLANK WITH HIP ROTATION
PLANK POSITION
FEET HOLDING THE BALL**

Primary muscles:
Transversus abdominis,
obliques, transversus
abdominis, multifidii

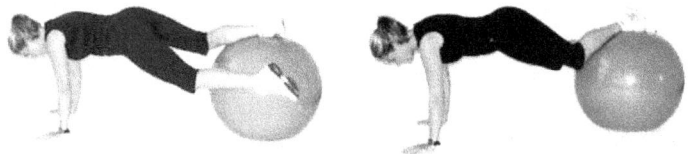

Supine on the floor. Shoulders and upper back on the floor. Heels on the ball. Contract the buttocks and hamstrings and lift the body into bridge position. Walk on the ball with the feet pressing down into the stability ball.	Contract the core muscles to stabilize. Keep the hips level.	Different arm position.
Supine on the floor. Upper back on the floor. One lower leg on the ball, the other leg to the side off the ball. Contract the buttocks and lift the body into bridge position. Hold the position or lower. Repeat. After a set repeat with the opposite leg.	Contract the core muscles to stabilize. Keep the hips level.	Different arm/leg position. Start from bridge position and lower one leg to the side. With or without hip rotation.
Supine on the floor. Upper back on the floor. Body in bridge position. Legs straight and together. Lower legs on the ball. Arm position optional. Contract the obliques, so the hips and legs rotate to one side. Repeat to the other side.	For intermediate exercisers. Contract the core muscles to stabilize. Keep the legs together and the body on a long straight line, then it is easier to keep the balance.	Different arm position.
Plank position. Hands on the floor. Lower legs are on each side of the ball, squeezing it. Contract the obliques, so the hips and legs rotate to one side. Hold the position – or slowly rotate, side to side. Repeat to the other side.	For advanced exercisers. Contract the core muscles to stabilize. Neck in neutral position. Watch the wrists. The wrists should be strengthened gradually.	Different arm position.

**TORSO ROTATION
ON ALL FOURS (THREE)
ON THE FLOOR
SUPPORTED BY BALL**

Primary muscles:
Rotators, multifidii,
erector spinae

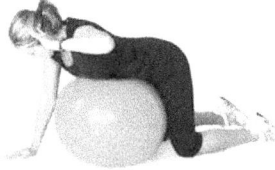

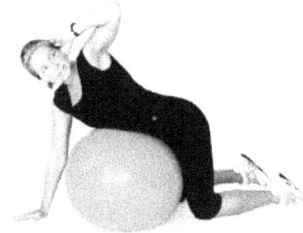

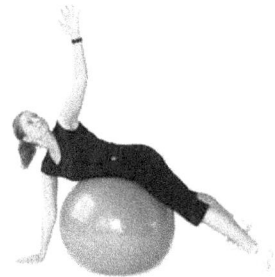

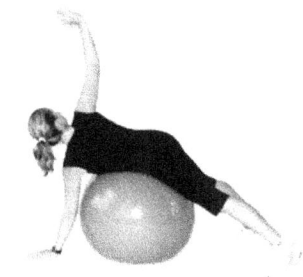

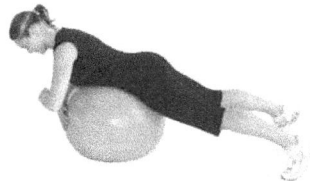

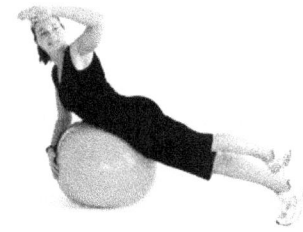

**TORSO ROTATION
PRONE ON THE BALL**

Primary muscles:
Rotators, multifidii,
erector spinae

**TORSO ROTATION
HAND ON BALL
PRONE ON THE BALL**

Primary muscles:
Rotators, multifidii,
erector spinae

**TORSO ROTATION
WITH ARM AND LEG LIFT
HAND ON BALL
PRONE ON THE BALL**

Primary muscles: Rotators,
multifidii, erector spinae,
gluteus maximus, hamstrings

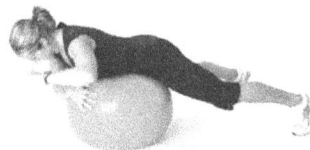

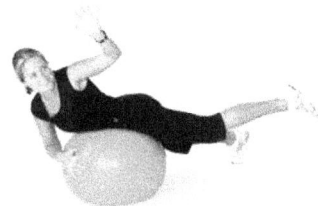

On all fours supported by the ball. Legs bent, lower legs on the floor. One hand on the floor. Opposite hand by the head. Lift the torso and rotate to one side, while the the elbow lifts towards the ceiling. Lower the torso. Repeat. After a set repeat to the opposite side.	For beginners. Contract the core muscles to stabilize. Neck in neutral position.	Different arm position.
Prone on the ball. Feet on the floor. Hands on the floor. Rotate the torso. The top arm moves up to open up the chest. Look to the top hand. Return. Lower the arm. Repeat or repeat to the opposite side.	Contract the core muscles to stabilize. Neck in neutral position.	Different arm position. Different leg position: The feet can be wide apart or together.
Prone on the ball. Feet on the floor. One hand on the ball, other arm to the side or by the head. Lift and rotate the torso to one side, free arm lifts to the ceiling. Look to the arm Lower the body. Repeat to the same side. After a set, repeat opposite.	For intermediate exercisers. Contract the core muscles to stabilize. Neck in neutral position. Complete a set to one side, then the hands change place, complete a set to the other side.	Different arm position: The arms can be by the side, the hands under the forehead, behind the head or to the side. Different leg position: The feet can be wide apart or together.
Prone on the ball. Feet on the floor. One hand on the stability ball, other hand lifted, free. Lift and rotate the torso to the side, lift the arm upwards. Look to the hand. At the same time lift the leg at the same side. Lower the arm, torso and leg. Repeat.	For advanced exercisers. Challenging balance work. Contract the core muscles to stabilize. Neck in neutral position. Complete a set to one side, then the hands change place, complete a set to the other side.	Different arm position: Different leg position: The feet can be wide apart or together.

**BACK EXTENSION
WITH ROTATION
PRONE ON THE BALL**

Primary muscles:
Erector spinae, rotators,
multifidii

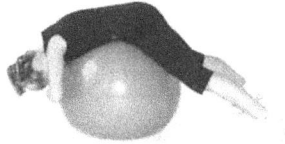

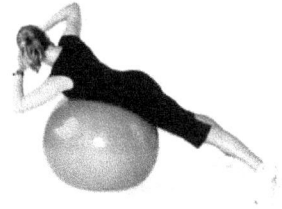

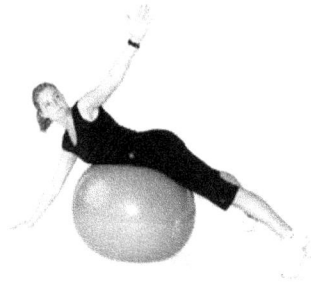

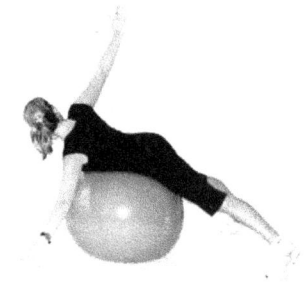

**AIRPLANE
PRONE ON THE BALL**

Primary muscles:
Erector spinae, rotators,
multifidii

**DIVE (PREPARATION)
PRONE ON THE BALL**

Primary muscles:
Gluteus maximus, hamstrings,
erector spinae, deltoids

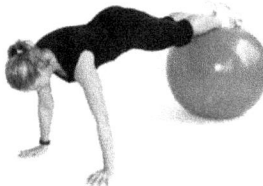

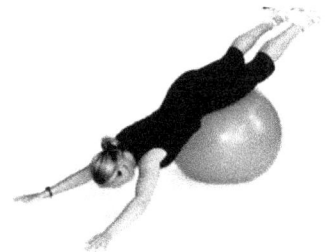

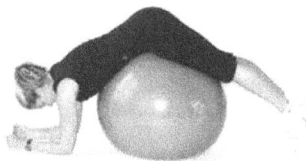

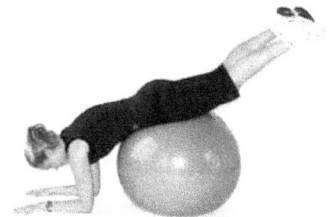

**HIP EXTENSION
(GOLD FISH)
PRONE ON THE BALL**

Primary muscles:
Gluteus maximus, hamstrings,
erector spinae

Prone on the ball. Feet on the floor. Arm position optional. Lift and rotate the torso to one side. Return and lower the torso all the way down. Repeat other side.	Contract the core muscles to stabilize. Neck in neutral position.	Different arm position: The arms can be by the side, the hands under the forehead, behind the head or to the side. Different leg position: The feet can be wide apart or together.
Prone on the ball. Feet are the floor. Arms to the side. The hands do not touch the floor. Contract the back extensors and lift the torso. Hold. In this position rotate the torso from side to side.	Contract the core muscles to stabilize. Neck in neutral position. Keep the spine in neutral position. This makes it easier to rotate.	Different arm position: The arms can be by the side, the hands under the forehead, behind the head or to the side. Different leg position: The feet can be wide apart or together.
Plank. Lower legs on ball. Hands on the floor directly below the shoulders. Body in a straight line. The arms push the body backwards, so the torso dives down and the legs go up. The arms pull and bring the body back into horizontal position.	Contract the core muscles to stabilize. Neck in neutral position.	Different arm/leg position. Different range of motion.
Prone on the ball. Forearms or hands on the floor. Legs together and down – the toes do *not* touch the floor. Contract the buttocks and lift the legs high into hip extension. Lower the legs with control.	Contract the core muscles to stabilize. Neck in neutral position. In the first part of the exercise focus on the buttocks and hamstrings, in the last part focus on the back extensors.	Different arm/leg position. Different range of motion.

BACK EXTENSION
KNEELING ON THE FLOOR
SUPPORTED BY THE BALL

Primary muscles:
Erector spinae,
gluteus maximus, hamstrings

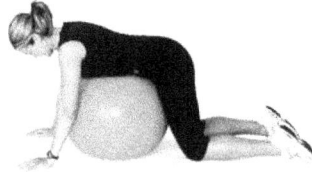

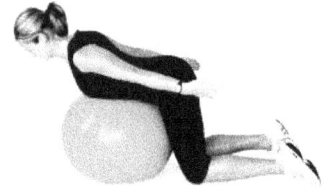

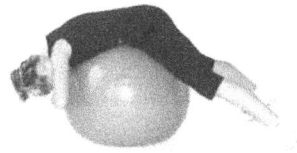

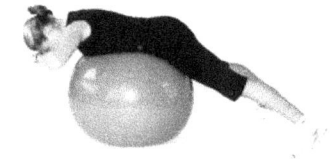

BACK EXTENSION
PRONE ON THE BALL

Primary muscles:
Erector spinae,
gluteus maximus, hamstrings

PARACHUTE JUMP
PRONE ON THE BALL

Primary muscles:
Erector spinae,
gluteus maximus, hamstrings,
transversus abdominis,
multifidii

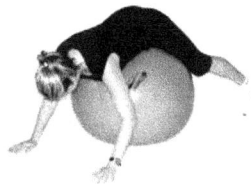

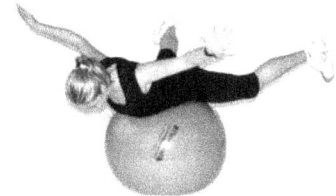

QUADRUPED
ON ALL FOURS ON FLOOR
SUPPORTED BY THE BALL

Primary muscles: Rotators,
multifidii, transversus
abdominis, hamstrings,
gluteus maximus, deltoids,

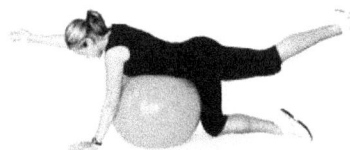

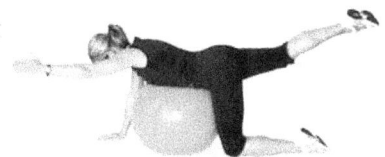

TECHNIQUE	BENEFIT	VARIATION
Kneeling. Lower legs on the floor. Torso supported by the ball. Hands on the floor in front of the ball or by the side. Contract the lower back and lift the torso and arms up into a back extension over the ball. Hold this position for a moment and lower. Repeat.	For beginners. A back extension with bent legs, lower legs on the floor. Contract the core muscles to stabilize. Neck in neutral position.	Different arm position. The top postion may be held isometrically while performing different arm movements.
Prone on the ball. Feet on the floor. Arm position is optional. Contract and lift the torso up into a back extension. Lower the torso. Repeat.	Contract the core muscles to stabilize. Neck in neutral position.	Different arm position: The arms can be by the side, the hands under the forehead, behind the head or forward (overhead). Different leg position: The feet can be wide apart or together.
Prone on the ball. Hands and toes on the floor. Lift the arms and legs from the floor up past horizontal and hold the position. Arms and legs out as in a 'parachute jump'. Contract all the muscles on the back side of the body to keep the limbs lifted and keep the balance.	For intermediate to advanced exercisers. An exercise for the entire back side of the body. Contract the core muscles to stabilize.	Different arm/leg position. Isometric or dynamic exercise.
On all fours, supported by the ball. Hands on the floor. Lift one arm and the opposite leg to horizontal. Lower. Repeat with the opposite arm and leg.	For beginners. For the small stabilizing muscles in the back. Free arm slightly to the side and thumb to the ceiling – to reduce stress on the shoulder. Contract the core to stabilize. Neck in neutral position.	Different arm/body/leg position. Repeat or alternate each time. **SAME SIDE ARM AND LEG LIFT** Lift the same side arm and leg at the same time. Alternate, change side.

**SUPERMAN
PRONE ON THE BALL**

Primary muscles:
Rotators, multifidii,
transversus abdominis,
hamstrings, gluteus maximus

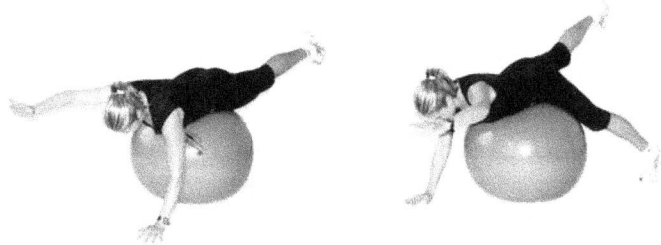

**SUPERMAN
SUPPORT HAND ON BALL
PRONE ON THE BALL**

Primary muscles: Rotators,
multifidii, transversus
abdominis, hamstrings, gluteus
maximus

**SUPERMAN
LEGS OFF THE FLOOR
PRONE ON THE BALL**

Primary muscles: Rotators,
multifidii, transversus
abdominis, hamstrings, gluteus
maximus, deltoids

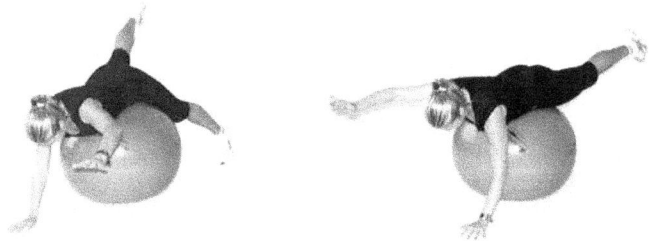

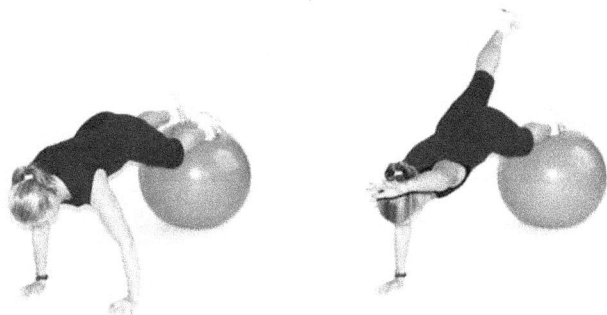

**SUPERMAN
PLANK POSITION
FEET ON THE BALL**

Primary muscles: Rotators,
multifidii, transversus
abdominis, hamstrings, gluteus
maximus, deltoids

Prone on the ball. Hands and toes on the floor. Lift one arm and the opposite leg above horizontal. Lower. Repeat with the opposite arm and leg. Note: Arm is forward and a little to the side with the thumb up.	Contract the core muscles to stabilize. Neck in neutral position. Excellent exercise for the small stabilizing muscles in the back. Initial progression: Lift arms alternatingly, while the legs are on the floor. Or: Lift the legs alternatingly, while the hands are on the floor.	Repeat exercise or alternate. 1. Lift the torso into back extension at the same time. 2. In top position lift the arm and leg to the side. 3. In top position touch the hand to the opposite foot. **SAME SIDE ARM/LEG LIFT** Same side arm and leg lift at the same time. Change side.
Prone on the ball. Lift one arm forward and up and at the same time lift the opposite leg to horizontal. In stead of supporting the hand on the floor, put the arm on the the ball. Repeat with the opposite arm and leg.	For intermediate exercisers. Contract the core muscles to stabilize. Neck in neutral position.	Different arm/leg position. The torso may lift into a back extension at the same time.
Prone on the ball. Hands on the floor. Legs down, but the toes do not touch the floor. Lift one arm and the opposite leg above horizontal. Lower. Repeat with the opposite arm and leg.	For advanced exercisers. Contract the core muscles to stabilize. Neck in neutral position.	Different arm/leg position. Repeat exercise or alternate.
Plank position. Feet or lower legs on the ball. Hands on the floor. Contract the core and keep the body in a straight line. Lift one leg and the opposite arm. Lower. Repeat with the opposite arm and leg.	For very advanced exercisers. A moderate tempo is recommended, not too fast, not too slow.	Different point of support.

PLANK, FLEXED HIPS
FOREARMS ON THE BALL
LOWER LEGS ON THE FLOOR

Primary muscles:
Transversus abdominis,
multifidii

PLANK
FOREARMS ON THE BALL

Primary muscles:
Transversus abdominis,
multifidii, deltoids

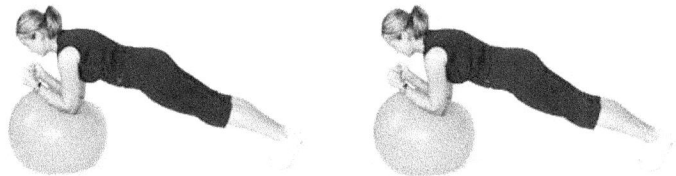

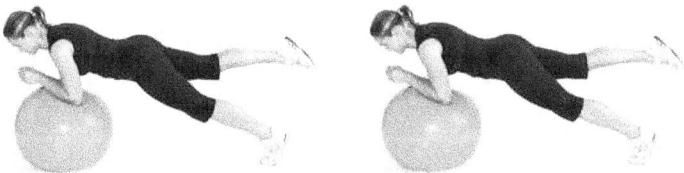

PLANK, ONE LEG LIFTED
FOREARMS ON THE BALL

Primary muscles:
Transversus abdominis,
multifidii, deltoids

PLANK
ONE FOREARM ON THE BALL

Primary muscles:
Transversus abdominis,
multifidii, rotators,
gluteus maximus, hamstrings

On all fours behind the ball. The arms are bent, forearms are on top of the ball. Contract the core muscles to stabilize. Hold the position.	Contract the core muscles to stabilize. Keep breathing.	Different arm/body position. Different degree af hip flexion. With one forearm on the stability ball, the other arm free, lifted forward off the ball (for advanced exercisers).
Plank position. Forearms on top of the stability ball. Feet on the floor. Contract the core muscles to stabilize. The body is in a straight line. Hold the position.	For intermediate exercisers. Contract the core muscles to stabilize. Neck in neutral position. Keep breathing.	Different arm/body/leg position.
Plank position. Forearms on top of the stability ball. One foot on the floor, the free leg is lifted. The hips are level. Contract the core muscles to stabilize. The body is in a straight line. Hold the position.	For intermediate exercisers. Contract the core muscles to stabilize. Neck in neutral position. Hips are level. Keep breathing.	Different arm/body/leg position.
Plank position. One forearm on top of the ball. The free arm is forward, to the side or on the back. Toes on the floor. Contract the core muscles to stabilize and keep the body in a straight line. Hold the position.	For advanced exercisers. Contract the core muscles to stabilize. Neck in neutral position. Hips are level. Keep breathing.	Different arm/body position.

**PLANK
ON ALL FOURS,
KNEES OFF THE FLOOR
FOREARMS ON THE BALL**

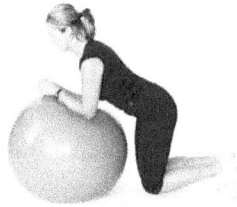

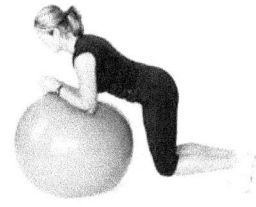

Primary muscles:
Transversus abdominis,
multifidii, obliques, deltoids

**PLANK WITH LEG LIFT
ON ALL FOURS,
KNEES OFF THE FLOOR
FOREARMS ON THE BALL**

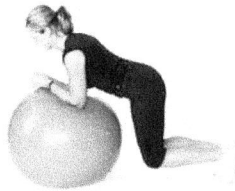

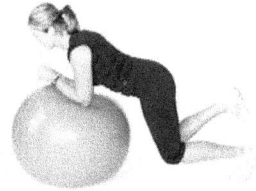

Primary muscles:
Transversus abdominis,
multifidii, rotators

**PLANK (PRONE BRIDGE)
THIGHS ON THE BALL**

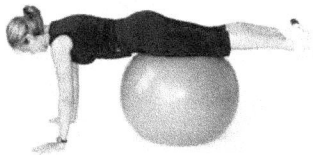

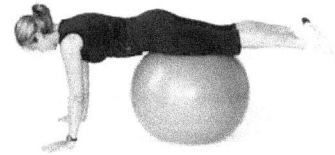

Primary muscles:
Transversus abdominis,
multifidii, deltoids

**PLANK PULL
(PRONE BRIDGE PULL)
THIGHS ON THE BALL**

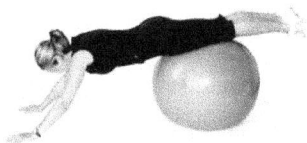

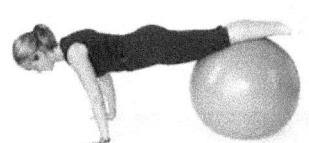

Primary muscles:
Transversus abdominis,
multifidii, latissimus dorsi,
deltoids

On all fours behind the ball. Toes on the floor. The arms are bent, forearms are on top of the ball. Contract the core to stabilize. Lift the knees approximately ½ inch, 1 cm, off the floor. Hold the position.	Contract the core muscles to stabilize. Keep breathing.	Different arm position. Different leg position. Press the thighs together to activate the adductors. Hold the position with or without movement of the legs, eg. lifting and lowering the knees to the floor.
On all fours behind the ball. Toes on the floor. The arms are bent, forearms are on top of the ball. Contract the core to stabilize. Lift the knees lifts approx. ½ inch, 1 cm, off the floor. Hold the position. Lift one leg. Keep the hips level. Lower and repeat opposite.	Contract the core to stabilize. Keep pelvis in neutral position, when lifting the leg. Keep breathing.	Different leg position.
Plank position. Thighs on top of the stability ball. Hands on the floor. Contract the core muscles to stabilize. The body is in a straight line. Hold the position.	Contract the core to stabilize. Neck in neutral position. Keep breathing. This position can be hard on the wrists. The wrists should be strengthened gradually with few repetitions initially, short lever, more rest between sets.	Different arm/body/leg position. On the thighs, lower legs or the toes (easy to hard).
Plank position. Thighs on top of the ball. Hands on the floor in front of the shoulders. Contract the back muscles and pull the arms back and under the torso, so the body rolls forward on the ball. Push the body backwards again. Repeat.	Isometric exercise for the core. Dynamic for the back and the shoulders. Neck in neutral position. This position can be hard on the wrists. The wrists should be strengthened gradually with few repetitions initially, short lever, more rest between sets.	Different range of motion.

PLANK
(PRONE BRIDGE)
TOES ON THE BALL

Primary muscles:
Transversus abdominis,
multifidii, deltoids

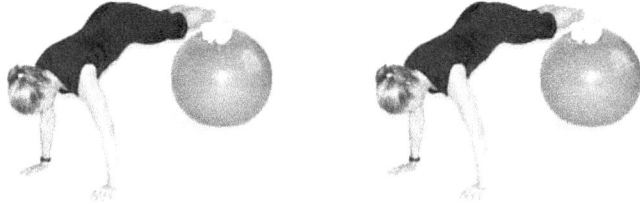

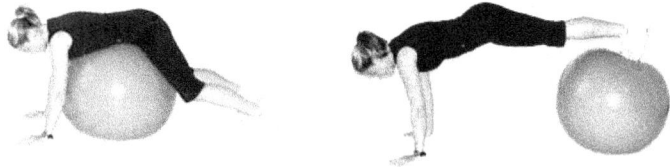

WALK OUT
PLANK POSITION

Primary muscles:
Transversus abdominis,
multifidii, deltoids

PLANK WITH LEGPULL
PLANK POSITION,
LOWER LEGS ON THE BALL

Primary muscles:
Transversus abdominis,
multifidii, quadriceps,
iliopsoas, deltoids

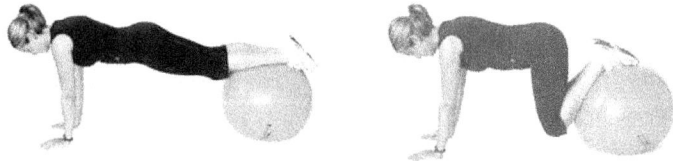

PLANK MARCH ON TOP
PLANK POSITION
TOES ON THE BALL

Primary muscles:
Transversus abdominis,
gluteus maximus, hamstrings,
multifidii, deltoids

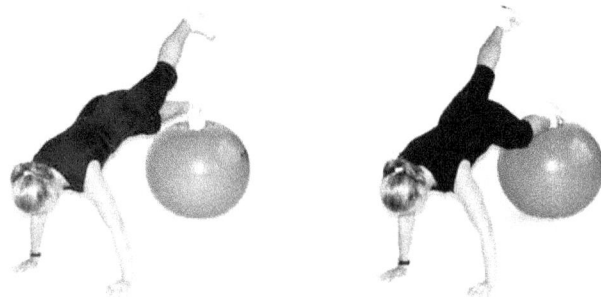

TECHNIQUE	NOTE	VARIATION
Plank position. Hands on the floor. Feet, toes, on top of the stability ball. Contract the core muscles to stabilize the body. The body is in a straight line. Hold the position.	Contract the core muscles to stabilize. Neck in neutral position. Keep breathing. This position can be hard on the wrists. The wrists should be strengthened gradually with few repetitions initially, short lever, more rest between sets.	Different arm position. With both or one leg on the ball.
Prone on the ball. Contract the core muscles to stabilize. The body is on a straight line. Walk forward with the hands as far as you can, until you are on your lower legs or toes. Hold this position for a moment or walk backwards with the hands to the starting position.	Moderate tempo. Control the movement – especially on the return trip; the ball often starts to roll. This position can be hard on the wrists. The wrists should be strengthened gradually with few repetitions initially, short lever, more rest between sets.	Different point of support. End range of motion on the thighs, lower legs, ankle or the toes (easy to hard).
Plank position. Hands on the floor shoulder-width apart. Lower legs on top of the stability ball. The body is in a straight line. Bend the legs, knees stop right above the floor. Straigthen the legs, return to plank position.	Contract the core muscles to stabilize. Neck in neutral position. Moderate tempo. This position can be hard on the wrists. The wrists should be strengthened gradually with few repetitions initially, short lever, more rest between sets.	Different arm position.
Plank position. Hands on the floor shoulder-width apart. Feet, toes, on top of the stability ball. Contract the core muscles and keep the body in a straight line. Lift one leg at a time, walk with the toes on top of the ball.	For advanced exercisers. Contract the core muscles to stabilize. Neck in neutral position. Keep breathing. This position can be hard on the wrists. The wrists should be strengthened gradually with few repetitions initially, short lever, more rest between sets.	Different arm position.

PLANK **FEET ON THE BALL** **SUPPORT ON ONE ARM** Primary muscles: Transversus abdominis, multifidii, deltoids	
PLANK TORSO ROTATION **(PRONE BALL ROLL)** **PRONE ON THE BALL** Primary muscles: Transversus abdominis, multifidii, obliques externus and internus	
PLANK **WITH HIP ROTATION** **FEET HOLDING THE BALL** Primary muscles: Transversus abdominis, multifidii, rotators, obliques externus and internus, deltoids	
PLANK CRAWL **(PRONE CRAWLER)** Primary muscles: Transversus abdominis, multifidii, deltoids, latissimus dorsi	

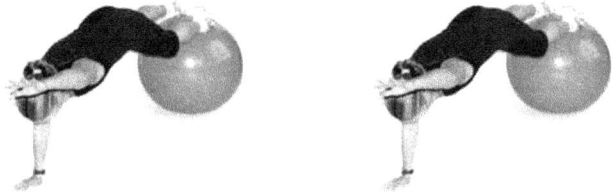

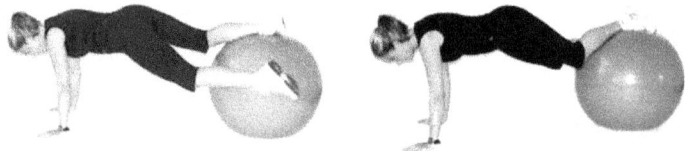

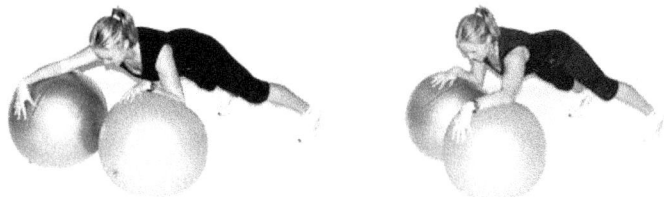

Plank position. Feet, toes, on the ball. One hand is on the floor, the free arm is in an optional position. Contract the core muscles to stabilize. Hold the position (the arm can move). After a while change to the opposite arm.	For advanced exercisers. Contract the core muscles to stabilize. Neck in neutral position. Isometric exercise. Keep breathing.	Different arm/leg position. The free arm can be lifted forward, outward, backward, in a circle or different patterns.
Prone on the ball. Arms around the ball. Feet wide apart on the floor. Rotate the torso, so the body and the ball roll from side to side.	For intermediate exercisers. Contract the core muscles to stabilize. Relax the head and the neck.	Different leg position. **PRONE BALL ROLL WITH LEG CHANGE** Roll to the side. The leg at the opposite side lifts. Change side.
Plank position. Hands on the floor. Lower legs are on each side of the ball squeezing it tightly. Contract the obliques to rotate the hips, legs and ball from side to side.	For advanced exercisers. Contract the core muscles to stabilize. Neck in neutral position.	Different arm/leg position.
Plank position. Two balls. Arms bent. One forearm on each ball. Feet on the floor. Contract the core muscles to stabilize the body. The arms pull alternatingly towards the body in a crawling movement.	For advanced exercisers. Contract the core muscles to stabilize. Neck in neutral position. Keep breathing.	Different leg position. **SUPINE CRAWLER** For advanced exercisers. (Paul Chek) Two balls. Bridge position with one bent arm on each ball. The arms pull alternatingly in a crawling movement, while contracting the back and core.

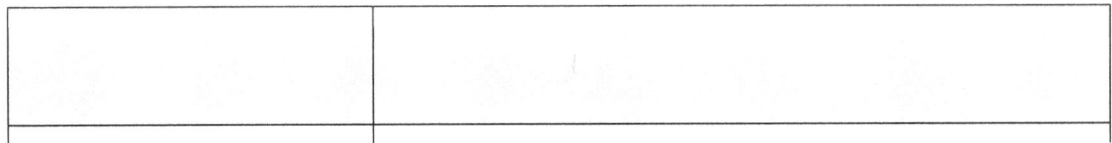

HEEL RAISE
SITTING ON THE BALL

Primary muscles:
Transversus abdominis,
multifidii, erector spinae,
soleus

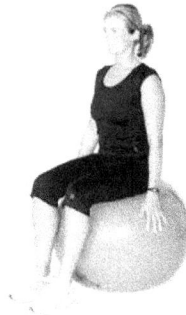

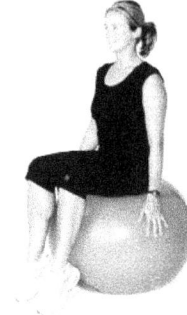

PELVIC TILT
(WITH/WITHOUT SUPPORT)
SITTING ON THE BALL

Primary muscles:
Transversus abdominis,
multifidii, rectus abdominis,
erector spinae

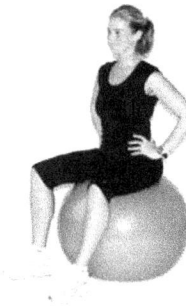

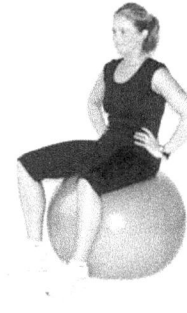

PELVIC SIDE TILT
(WITH/WITHOUT SUPPORT)
SITTING ON THE BALL

Primary muscles:
Transversus abdominis,
multifidii, obliques

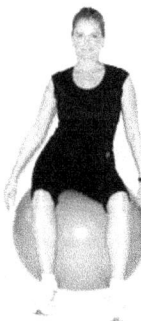

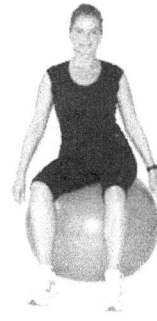

HIP CIRCLES
(WITH/WITHOUT SUPPORT)
SITTING ON THE BALL

Primary muscles:
Transversus abdominis,
multifidii, obliques externus
and internus

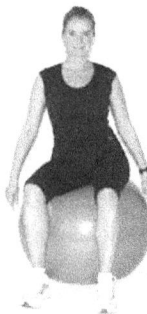

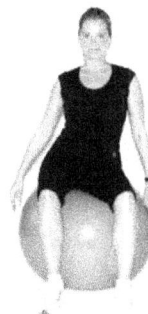

Sitting on the ball. The arms are down by the side, at the waist or to the side. The feet are on the floor. Lift the heels. Lower the heels. Contract the core muscles to stabilize.	For beginning exercisers. Easy balance exercise. Contract the core muscles to stabilize. Neck in neutral position.	Different arm/body exercises. Raise the heels or the toes. One or both eyes closed.
Sitting on the ball. The arms are down by the side, at the waist or to the side. The feet are on the floor or lifted off the floor. Contract the core muscles to stabilize. Contract the abs and lower back muscles; tilt the pelvis forward and backward (sagittal plane movement).	Excellent specific warm-up and lower back mobility exercise. Contract the core muscles to stabilize. Neck in neutral position.	Different arm/body exercises. **PELVIC TWIST (TRANSVERSAL PLANE)** Keep the hips level and move one hipbone slightly in front of the other and return. Repeat opposite side. A very small movement.
Sitting on the ball. The arms are down by the side, at the waist or to the side. The feet are on the floor or lifted off the floor. Contract the core muscles to stabilize. Contract the obliques and rock the pelvis from side to side (frontal plane movement).	Excellent specific warm-up and lower back mobility exercise. Contract the core muscles to stabilize. Neck in neutral position.	Different arm/leg position.
Sitting on the ball. The arms are down by the side, at the waist or to the side. The feet are on the floor or lifted off the floor Move the hips from side to side and forward and back in a circular movement. Repeat the opposite way.	Excellent specific warm-up and lower back mobility exercise. Contract the core muscles to stabilize. Neck in neutral position.	Different arm/leg position. **FIGURE EIGHT** Keep the torso stable and make figure eights – or infinity symbols – with the hips. Repeat the opposite way

7 | Lower Body Exercises

In this section you find lower body exercises, for the hips, legs and lower legs, with the stability ball, for one exerciser and one ball. In most of the exercises you also work the core muscles.

The exercise are categorized after primary muscles and muscle group and roughly 'from top to toe', not necessarily in the recommended sequence for a workout.

There is a wide selection of exercises and you have to make your own decision as to which exercise is best for your purpose.

Some exercises are very easy, some very difficult. In some cases there is a note explaining if it is an easy or difficult exercise, but not in all cases as many factors play a role.

Therefore some knowledge of sports science is necessary in order to be able to select the right exercise for a given exerciser.

Most exercises can be varied by using one or both arms or legs and by changing the arm-, body- or leg position.

The point of support can be changed, eg. from the hips to the thighs to the lower legs, ankles or toes. This results in a marked increase of the load on the muscles.

Most exercises can be made more difficult by increasing the balance work via decreasing the base of support, eg. from sitting on the ball with the feet wide apart to feet together or just one foot on the floor.

All the exercises can be changed, made easier or harder, by using balls of different sizes and degree of inflation.

Important: All exercises are for healthy exercisers free from any serious or disabilitating disease, illness or ailments. Please consult your doctor before beginning these exercises.

Muscles

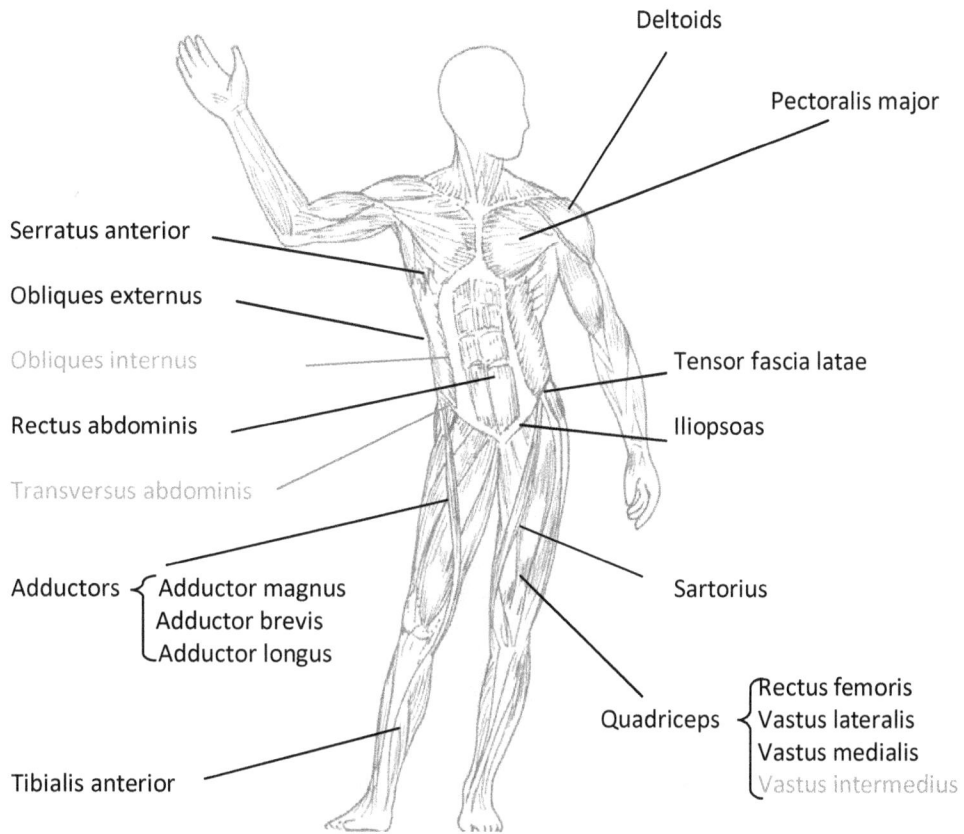

Deltoids

Pectoralis major

Serratus anterior

Obliques externus

Obliques internus

Rectus abdominis

Transversus abdominis

Tensor fascia latae

Iliopsoas

Adductors { Adductor magnus
Adductor brevis
Adductor longus

Sartorius

Quadriceps { Rectus femoris
Vastus lateralis
Vastus medialis
Vastus intermedius

Tibialis anterior

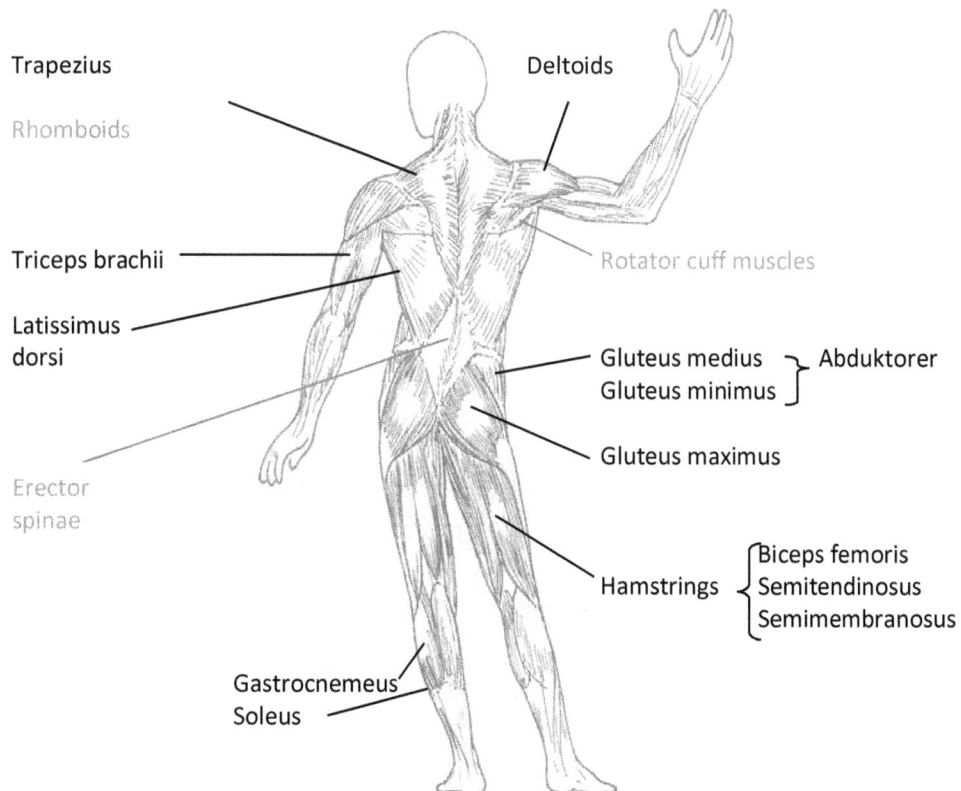

Trapezius

Rhomboids

Deltoids

Triceps brachii

Latissimus
dorsi

Rotator cuff muscles

Gluteus medius
Gluteus minimus } Abduktorer

Gluteus maximus

Erector
spinae

Biceps femoris
Semitendinosus
Semimembranosus

Hamstrings {

Gastrocnemeus
Soleus

**MARCH, WALK,
SITTING ON THE BALL**

Primary muscles:
Transversus abdominis,
multifidii,
iliopsoas, rectus femoris

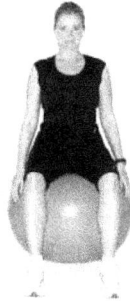

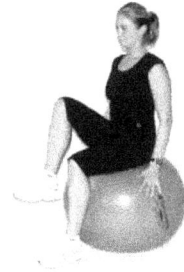

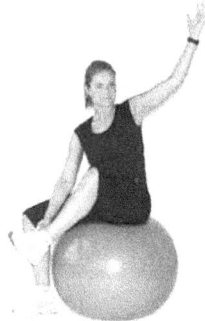

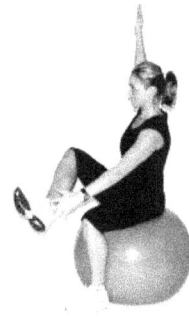

**LEG LIFT (ARM LIFT)
SITTING ON THE BALL**

Primary muscles:
Transversus abdominis,
multifidii,
iliopsoas, rectus femoris

**LEG LIFT/ARM LIFT (LOOK)
SITTING ON THE BALL**

Primary muscles:
Obliques externus and
internus, transversus
abdominis, multifidii,
iliopsoas, rectus femoris

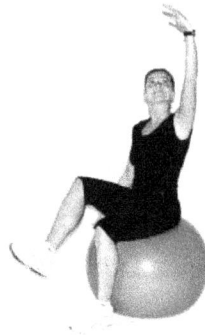

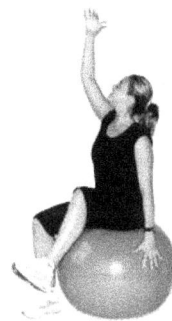

**OPPOSITE ARM/LEG LIFT
SEMI-SUPINE ON THE BALL**

Primary muscles:
Transversus abdominis, rectus
abdominis, obliques externus
and internus, multifidii,
iliopsoas, rectus femoris

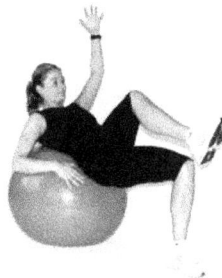

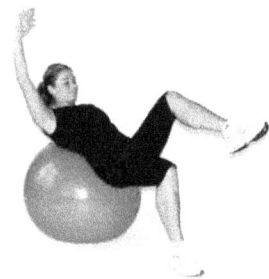

114

Sitting on the stability ball. Contract the core muscles to stabilize. The feet walk in place (or walk a full circle around the stability ball). The arms can be by the side or perform dynamic walking movements or various arm exercises.	Contract the core muscles to stabilize. Keep the torso erect. Neck in neutral position.	Arm position/exercise. **STEP TOUCH ON THE BALL** Sitting on the stability ball. Take a step from side to side. Side step and tap. Return. **DOUBLE STEP TOUCH** Sitting on the ball. Take two steps to the side, tap. Return.
Sitting on the stability ball. Feet on the floor. Lift one leg and touch the opposite hand to the foot. Lower. Repeat with the opposite leg.	Contract the core muscles to stabilize. Keep the torso erect. Neck in neutral position.	Different arm exercises. Or keep the arms by the side. With upper body movements – eg. torso rotation right and left.
Sitting on the stability ball. Lift the legs alternatingly; kneelift. Lift one leg and lift the opposite arm towards the ceiling. Lower. Repeat with the opposite leg and arm. For additional challenge: Rotate the head and look to the lifted hand.	Contract the core muscles to stabilize. Keep the torso erect. Moderate tempo.	Different arm exercises. Different leg exercises.
Semi-supine position. Lower back supported. Feet shoulder-width apart on the floor. The arms on the ball or the thighs. Lift one leg and the opposite arm. Lower arm and leg with control. Repeat with opposite leg and arm.	For intermediate exercisers. Contract the core muscles to stabilize. Neck in neutral position.	Different arm/leg position.

**SITTING ON THE BALL
UNSUPPORTED**

Primary muscles:
Transversus abdominis,
multifidii

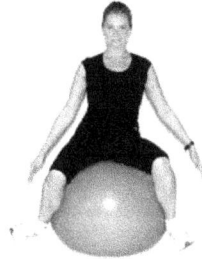

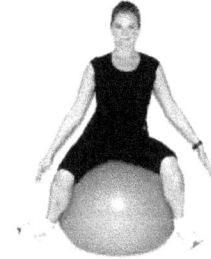

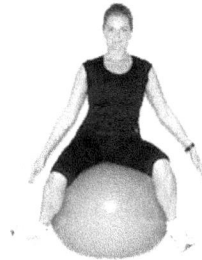

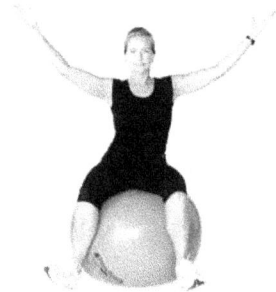

**SITTING ON THE BALL
UNSUPPORTED
WITH TORSO MOVEMENTS**

Primary muscles:
Transversus abdominis,
multifidii

**ON ALL FOURS
ON THE BALL**

Primary muscles:
Transversus abdominis,
multifidii, rectus abdominis

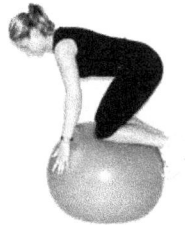

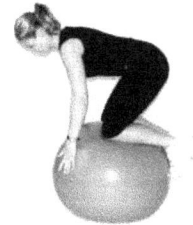

**ARM AND/OR LEG LIFT
ON ALL FOURS
ON THE BALL**

Primary muscles:
Transversus abdominis,
multifidii, rotators

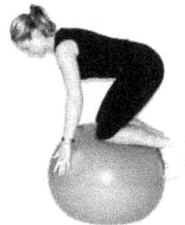

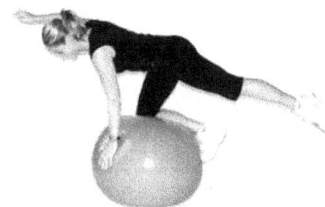

Sitting on the ball. Arms on the ball or to the side. The feet are lifted off the floor. The leg muscles contract to stabilize the body on the ball. Contract the core muscles to keep the balance.	Contract the core muscles to stabilize. Progression: Lift one foot at a time – and then both.	Different arm exercises. With upper body movements – eg. torso rotation right and left. Close one eye, then both eyes.
Sitting on the ball. The feet are lifted off the floor. The leg muscles contract to stabilize the body on the ball. Contract the core muscles to keep the balance. Perform arm and torso movements.	Contract the core muscles to stabilize.	Different arm exercises. With torso movement – eg. torso rotation right and left. Close one eye, then both eyes.
On all fours on the ball. Contract the core and leg muscles to stabilize the body on the ball. Keep the spine and neck in neutral position. Hold the position.	For intermediate exercisers. It is not all that difficult to keep the balance on the stability ball, but getting up there may require a little practice. Tip: Hold the ball firmly with the hands. Press the knees into the ball. Rock and roll back and forth and then hold. Keep breathing.	Different ball/ball inflation (affects the degree of difficulty, how much the ball rolls). Support on one or both legs.
On all fours on the ball. Contract the core and leg muscles to stabilize the body on the ball. Keep the spine and neck in neutral position. Hold the position. Lift one arm, lift one leg or lift one arm and the opposite leg. Repeat opposite side.	For intermediate exercisers. Progression: Lift one arm. Repeat opposite. Lift one leg. Repeat opposite. Lift arm and opposite leg. Repeat opposite side.	Different ball/ball inflation. Lift arm and/or leg up (sagittal plane) or to the side (frontal plane). Different arm/leg exercises.

KNEELING ON THE BALL

Primary muscles:
Transversus abdominis,
multifidii, erector spinae,
gluteus maximus, quadriceps

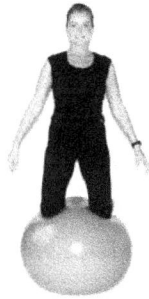

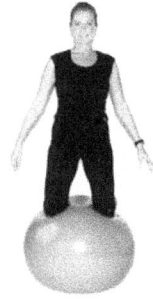

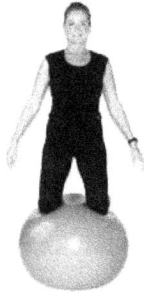

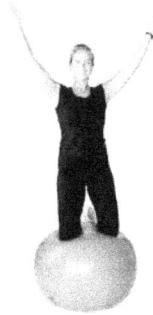

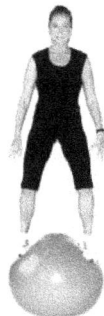

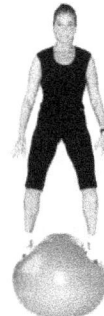

**KNEELING ON THE BALL
WITH TORSO MOVEMENTS**

Primary muscles:
Transversus abdominis,
multifidii, erector spinae,
gluteus maximus, quadriceps

STANDING ON THE BALL

Primary muscles:
Transversus abdominis,
multifidii, erector spinae,
gluteus maximus, quadriceps

SQUAT ON THE BALL

Primary muscles:
Transversus abdominis,
multifidii, erector spinae,
gluteus maximus, quadriceps,
gastrocnemeus, soleus

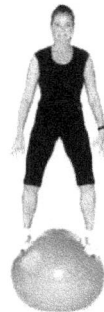

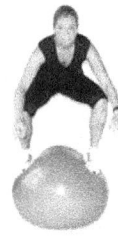

Kneeling on the ball. Contract the core and leg muscles to stabilize and keep the balance.	For intermediate exercisers. It is not that difficult to keep the balance on the knees on the stability ball, but getting up may require some practice. Tip: First get onto all fours, then go to upright. Get help from a partner or support yourself against a wallbar using both hands.	Different ball/ball inflation (affects the degree of difficulty, how much the ball rolls).
Kneeling on the ball. Contract the core and leg muscles to stabilize and keep the balance. Perform arm and torso movements for a more challenging workout.	For intermerdiate exercisers. Concentrate. It is not that difficult to keep the balance on the knees on the stability ball, but getting up may requires some practice. Tip: First get onto all fours, then go to upright. Get help from a partner or Support against a wallbar.	Different ball/ball inflation (affects the degree of difficulty, how much the ball rolls). Different upper body exercises – eg. torso rotation. With or without resistance.
Standing on the ball. Focus! Contract the core and leg muscles to stabilize and keep the balance. Keep contracting. Perform arm and torso movements for a more challenging workout.	For advanced exercisers. Concentrate. High risk. It is not that difficult to keep the balance standing on the ball, but getting up requires focus. Hold the ball firmly with the hands. Put one foot up, a little to the side, then the other. Find your balance and straighten the legs with control.	Different ball/ball inflation. Different upper body exercises. Get a partner to help you a couple of times or support yourself by a wall bar.
Standing on the ball. Focus! Contract the core and leg muscles to stabilize and keep the balance. Bend the legs into a squat and extend back up again. Start with a small range of motion. Increase ROM as you improve.	For advanced exercisers. Concentrate. High risk. It is not that difficult to keep the balance standing on the ball, but getting up requires focus. Hold the ball firmly with the hands. Put one foot up, a little to the side, then the other. Find your balance and straighten the legs with control	Different ball/ball inflation. Different arm/leg position. With or without resistance. You may perform the squat with a barbell or dumbbells, however the risk of injury is high. Is it worth the risk?

**BULGARIAN SQUAT
(SPLIT SQUAT)
FRONT FOOT ON FLOOR**

Primary muscles:
Quadriceps, gluteus maximus,
hamstrings, transversus
abdominis, multifidii

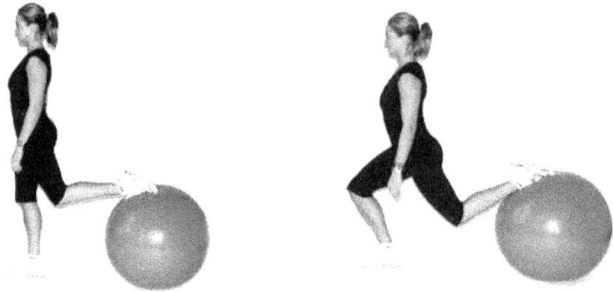

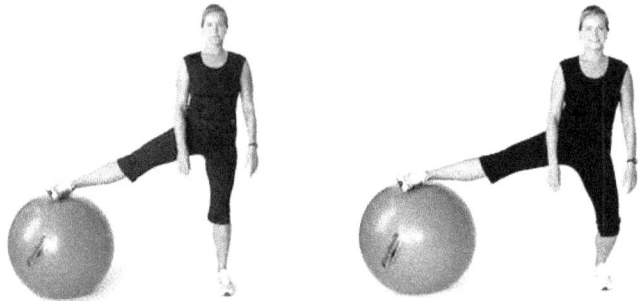

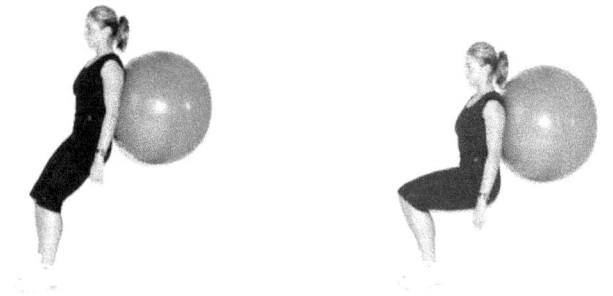

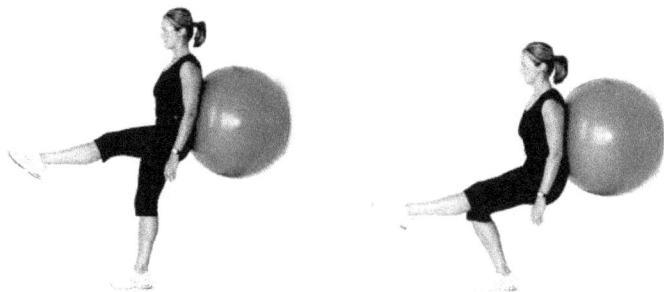

**SQUAT ONE LEG
(LATERAL ONE LEG SQUAT)
FREE LEG ON THE BALL**

Primary muscles:
Quadriceps, gluteus maximus,
hamstrings, transversus
abdominis, multifidii

**WALL SQUAT
(BACK WALL SLIDE)
STANDING ON THE FLOOR**

Primary muscles:
Quadriceps, gluteus maximus,
hamstrings, transversus
abdominis, multifidii

**WALL SQUAT, ONE LEG
(ONE LEG WALL SQUAT)**

Primary muscles:
Quadriceps, gluteus maximus,
hamstrings, transversus
abdominis, multifidii

Standing. One foot firmly on the ground. The other leg is extended backward. The foot, toes, is on top of the stability ball. Bend the front leg into a one-leg squat. Extend the leg. Repeat. After a set repeat with the opposite leg.	Knee and foot must be aligned, no rotation of the knees. The front lower leg is close to vertical in the end position. Requires some hip flexor and adductor flexibility. For balance work.	Different arm/leg position. Range of motion, degree of knee flexion. With the front the foot on a BOSU, balance pillow, therapy trainer, teeterboard or other balance equipment.
Standing. One foot firmly on the ground. The other leg is abducted to the side. The lower leg, side of the foot, is on the ball. Bend the supporting leg into a one-leg squat. Extend the leg. Repeat. After a set repeat with the opposite leg.	Knee and foot must be aligned, no rotation of the knees. Requires flexible adductors.	**SQUAT AND ADDUCTION** Squat. When extending the supporting leg, adduct and bend the leg on the ball. Squat, extend leg, roll ball back out. **SQUAT AND HIP WORK** For hip mobility the exercise may include circles and patterns with the leg on the ball (Juan Carlos Santana)
Standing. Feet on the floor. Back to the wall. Lower back on the stability ball pressed against the wall. Lean the body back into the stability ball and perform a squat. Extend the legs and move back up.	Knees must be aligned with the feet, no rotation of the knees. Moderate tempo. Starting position is with the stability ball, middle part, at navel level.	With one or both legs.
Standing. One foot on the floor. Other leg is lifted off the floor in front of the body. Back to the wall. Lower back on the stability ball pressed against the wall. Lean the body back into the stability ball and perform a one-leg squat. Extend the leg and go back up.	Contract the core muscles to stabilize. Keep the hips level. Starting position is with the stability ball, middle part, at navel level.	Different arm position. Different position of the free leg, bent or straight forward as in pistols/stork pres. For advanced exercisers.

WALL SIT
STANDING ON THE FLOOR

Primary muscles:
Quadriceps, gluteus maximus,
hamstrings, transversus
abdominis, multifidii

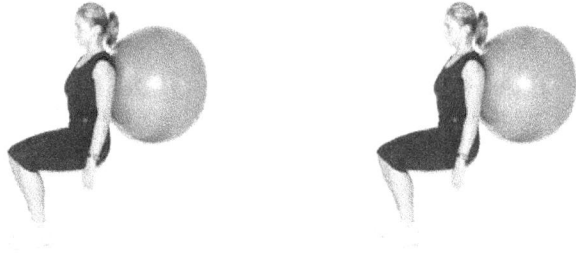

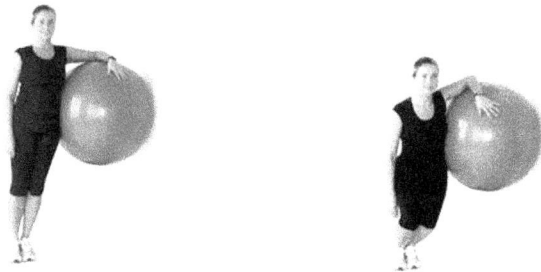

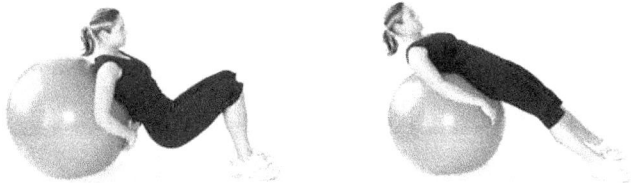

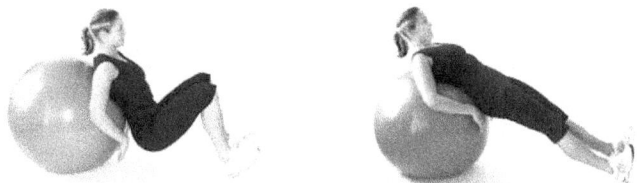

LATERAL WALL SQUAT
(LATERAL WALL SLIDE)
STANDING ON THE FLOOR

Primary muscles:
Quadriceps, gluteus maximus,
hamstrings, transversus
abdominis, multifidii

LEG PRESS
SEMI-SUPINE

Primary muscles:
Quadriceps, gluteus maximus,
hamstrings, transversus
abdominis, multifidii

LEG PRESS ON THE HEELS
(LEGPRES, HEEL BALANCE)
SEMI-SUPINE

Primary muscles:
Quadriceps, gluteus maximus,
hamstrings, transversus
abdominis, multifidii

Standing. Feet shoulder-width apart. Back to the wall. Lower back on the stability ball pressed against the wall. Bend the legs to a parallel squat. Lean the body back into the stability ball, and hold the position.	Isometric exercise. Knees and feet must be aligned, no rotation of the knees.	Different arm/leg position. Range of motion; different degree of knee flexion.
Standing. Feet together. Side to the wall. Lean into the ball with the shoulder (on the photo the arm is on top of the ball, but it can be by the side). The body is at an angle to the wall, approx. 60 degrees. Bend the legs, squat. Extend the legs and return.	For intermediate exercisers. For special strength and mobility of the lower legs and ankles (Juan Carlos Santana, Stability ball Training).	Different arm/leg position.
Supine; a semi-supine position. Upper back on the ball. Legs are straight and feet are on the floor shoulder-width apart. Press the body into the stability ball to keep it in place under the body. Perform a legpress; bend and extend the legs.	Easy exercise. Be careful that the ball does not shoot out backwards. Contract the core to stabilize. Knees and feet must be aligned, no rotation of the knees. Moderate tempo.	With both legs or one leg (for advanced exercisers).
Supine; a semi-supine position. Upper back on the ball. Legs are straight and heels are on the floor shoulder-width apart. Press the body into the ball to keep it in place under the body. Perform a leg press; bend and extend the legs.	Easy exercise. Be careful that the ball does not shoot out backwards. Contract the core to stabilize. Knees and feet must be aligned, no rotation of the knees. Moderate tempo.	With both legs or one leg (for advanced exercisers).

**FRONT WALL SQUAT
(FRONT WALL SLIDE)
STANDING ON THE FLOOR**

Primary muscles:
Quadriceps, gluteus maximus,
hamstrings, transversus
abdominis, multifidii

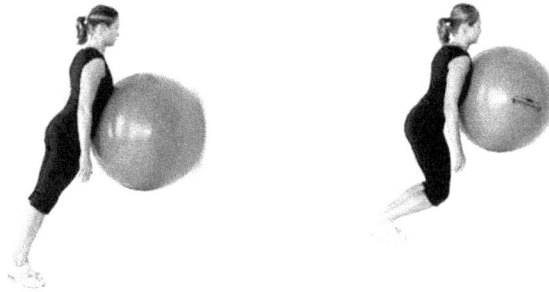

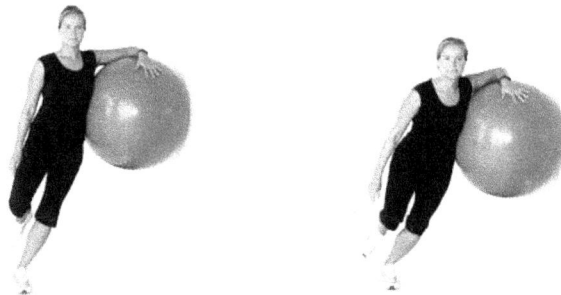

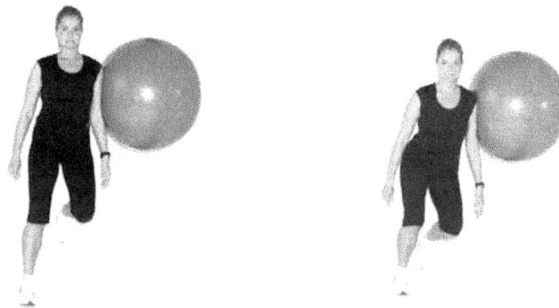

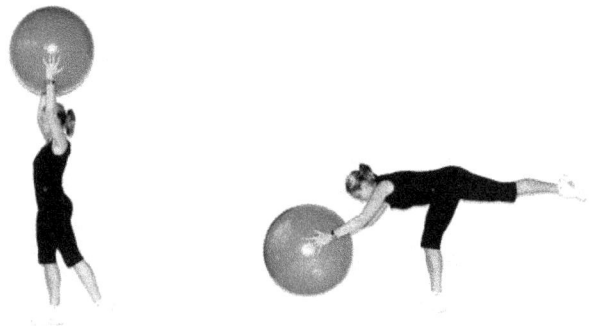

**LATERAL WALL SQUAT
STANDING, INSIDE LEG**

Primary muscles:
Quadriceps, gluteus maximus,
hamstrings, transversus
abdominis, multifidii

**LATERAL WALL SQUAT
STANDING, OUTSIDE LEG**

Primary muscles:
Quadriceps, gluteus maximus,
hamstrings, transversus
abdominis, multifidii

**ROMANIAN ONE-LEG
DEADLIFT
STANDING ON THE FLOOR**

Primary muscles:
Quadriceps, gluteus maximus,
hamstrings, transversus
abdominis, multifidii

Standing. Facing the wall. Lean torso against the ball, approx. 60-70 degree angle, and press ball against the wall. The arms are down by the side. The toes are on the floor, the heels are lifted. Bend the legs, squat down. Extend the legs, return.	For intermediate exercisers. Contract the core muscles to stabilize, so the ball does not upset the stomach. For stabilization and lower leg work (Juan Carlos Santana, Stability ball Training).	Different arm/leg position. With one leg lifted off the floor (for intermediate exercisers).
Standing. Side to the wall. Lean against the ball, arm on top of the ball, so the body is at an angle to the wall, approx. 60-70 degree. Lift the outside leg and bend into a one-leg squat on the inside leg. Extend the leg and return. Repeat. After a set repeat opposite.	For intermediate exercisers to advanced exercisers. Perform with both the right and the left leg. Inside arm is forward on the ball or down. Outside arm is down or to the side for balance.	Different arm position.
Standing. Side to the wall. Lean against the ball, arm down by the side, so the body is at an angle to the wall, approx. 60-70 degree. Lift the inside leg and bend into a one-leg squat on the outside leg. Extend the leg and return. Repeat. After a set repeat opposite.	For intermediate exercisers to advanced exercisers. Perform with borh the right and the left leg. Inside arm is forward on the ball or down. Outside arm is down or to the side for balance.	Different arm position.
Standing on one leg, foot firmly on the ground. Other other leg is extended back. The arms hold the ball in front of the body or overhead. Tip the body forward into a T-balance. Contract the buttocks and hamstrings and return to upright position. Repeat. After a set repeat opposite.	Excellent exercise for buttock, hamstring and balance work. Keep knee aligned with foot, no rotation in the knee. Do not lean forward or drop the head. Lower the torso as one unit and keep torso and free leg in line to form a T.	Different arm position. On both legs. With or without stability ball. Use a medicine ball for increased load.

**UNILATERAL LEG PRESS
SITTING ON THE BALL**

Primary muscles:
Iliopsoas, quadriceps,
transversus abdominis,
multifidii

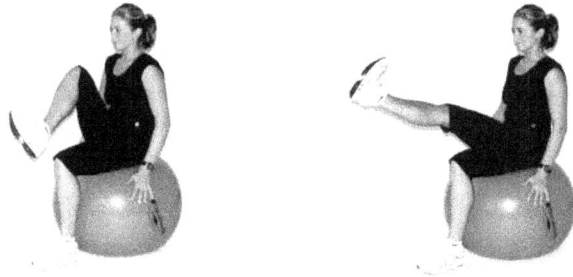

**KNEE EXTENSION
KNEELING ON THE FLOOR
WITH BALL SUPPORT**

Primary muscles:
Quadriceps, gluteus maximus,
hamstrings, transversus
abdominis

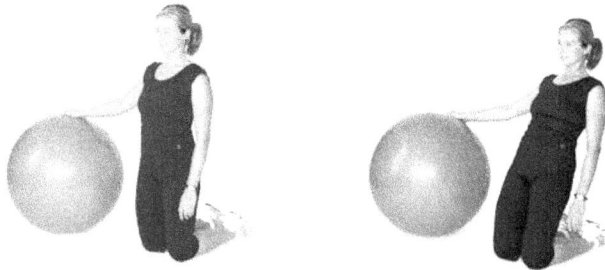

**SIDEPLANK EXTENSION
SITTING ON THE FLOOR TO
SIDELYING ON THE BALL**

Primary muscles:
Quadratus lumborum,
transversus abd., multifidii,
quadriceps, adductors

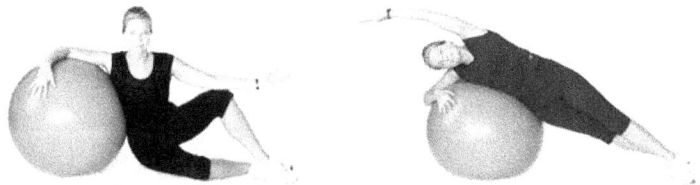

**STATIONARY 'NARROW'
LUNGE WITH BALL
STANDING ON THE FLOOR**

Primary muscles:
Quadriceps, gluteus maximus,
transversus abdominis,
multifidii

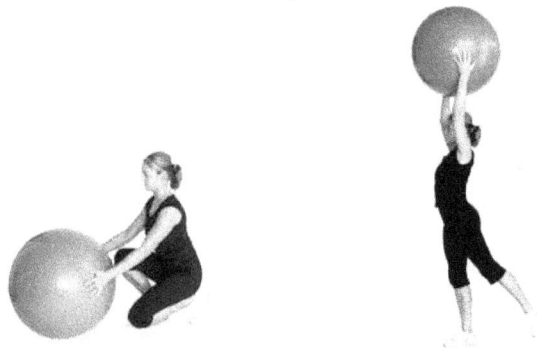

Sitting on the ball. Feet on the floor. Hands on the ball or to the side for balance. Kick one leg forward. Pull back. Repeat. After a set repeat opposite.	Contract the core muscles to stabilize.	Different arm/leg position. **LEG PRESS WITH ROTATION** The leg push straight forward at different angles, inward- or outward rotation.
Kneeling. The ball by the side of the body, one hand on top of the stability ball. Lower the body backward by bending the knees. Do not move at the hips. Extend the knees and return to upright position.	For intermediate to advanced exercisers. Not recommended for people with knee problems. Contract the core muscles to stabilize the torso well. Avoid arching the lower back.	Different arm position.
Sitting by the side of the ball. Both legs bent, bottom leg on the floor. Top foot on the floor in front of bottom foot. Inside arm is on the ball, the other is on the knee, palm up. Extend the hips and knees and roll sideways over the ball, side plank, with top arm overhead. Return with control	Pilates exercise with a ball. Contract the adductors and squeeze the legs together. Other pilates exercises may also be performed with the stability ball. Contract the core muscles to stabilize the body. After a set change side.	Different arm position.
Standing. Feet staggered. Back leg close behind the front leg, toes on the floor, heel lifted throughout the exercise. Arms overhead with the ball in the hands. Bend the legs into a 'narrow' stationary lunge. Extend back up. Repeat. After a set repeat with the opposite leg in front.	For intermediate exercisers. Perform with control, knees must be aligned with the feet; avoid rotation of the knees. Resistance exercise with an element of balance work. Contract the core muscles to stabilize.	Different range of motion. Arm variations. **LUNGES WITH BALL** Stationary lunges with ball. Lunge with ball. Sidelunge with ball. Lunge walk with ball. Lunge walk with torsorotation with ball.

**LUNGE BY THE BALL
FROM SITTING ON THE BALL**

Primary muscles:
Quadriceps, gluteus maximus,
hamstrings

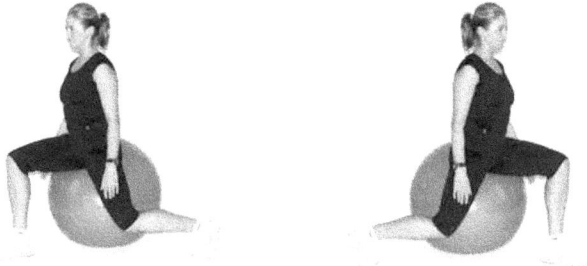

**HIP FLEXION WITH BALL
PLANK TO ONE LEG PLANK**

Primary muscles:
Iliopsoas, rectus femoris,
gluteus maximus, hamstrings,
transversus abd.is, multifidii

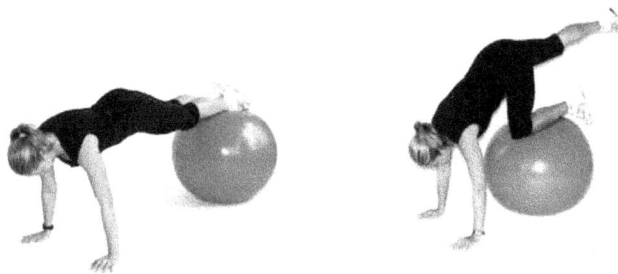

**HIP FLEXION
(SUPINE) BRIDGE POSITION
FOREARMS ON THE BALL**

Primary muscles:
Gluteus maximus, hamstrings,
iliopsoas, quadriceps,
transversus abd., multifidii

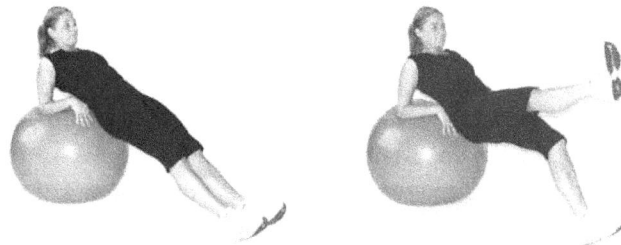

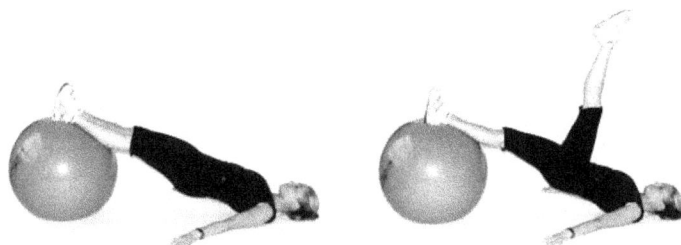

**HIP FLEXION
BRIDGE POSITION
FEET ON THE BALL**

Primary muscles:
Gluteus maximus, hamstrings,
iliopsoas, quadriceps,
transversus abd., multifidii

Sitting on the ball. Feet on the floor, legs together. Hop (or step) with a quarter turn into a lunge position with the side to the ball. Hop (or step) back into seated position. Hop (or step) with a quarter turn into a lunge the opposite way.	For intermediate to advanced exercisers. Requires coordination and muscular control. When jumping into lunge position, it is important to land in the right position, so hips, knees and feet are aligned.	Different arm position. Different leg position.
Plank position. One leg on the ball, other leg is slightly lifted off the ball. Hands on the floor. Pull the supporting leg towards the torso (hip and knee flexion), while pressing into the ball to create resistance. The free leg is passive, neutral. Return. Repeat. After a set repeat opposite.	For intermediate exercisers. Contract the core to stabilize. The free leg is in 'neutral', in the same position throughout the exercise. This position may be hard on the wrists. The wrists should be strengthened gradually.	Different arm position.
Bridge. Face away from the ball. The arms are bent, forearms on the ball. Legs are straight and feet, heels, are on the floor. Lift one leg, hip flexion. Lower. Repeat opposite.	For intermediate exercisers. For coordination, balance, stability, endurance and flexibility. Not hip strength. Contract the core muscles to stabilize.	Working leg bent or straight. Range of motion can be either small or large, a lift just above the floor or a high kick towards the torso.
Bridge on the floor. Lower legs on the ball. Arms on the floor. Upper back and shoulders on the floor. Lift one leg, hip flexion. Lower. Repeat with same leg or change leg.	Contract the core muscles to stabilize. Hips are level. For coordination, balance, stability, endurance and flexibility. Not hip strength. Requires some flexibility.	Working leg is bent or straight. Working leg may cross over the supporting leg or torso in a diagonal movement. Range of motion can be either small or large, a lift just above the ball or a high kick towards the torso.

KNEES PULL (SEA URCHIN)
PLANK POSITION
LOWER LEGS ON THE BALL

Primary muscles:
Rectus abdominis, obliques,
iliopsoas, quadriceps,
transversus abd., multifidii

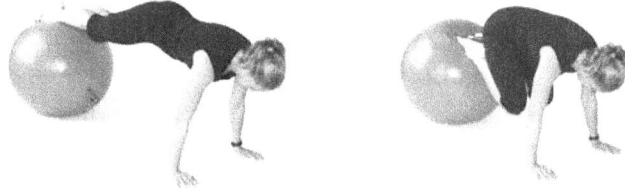

PLANK WITH
UNILATERAL BICYCLING
LOWER LEG ON BALL

Primary muscles:
Transversus abdominis,
multifidii, iliopsoas, quads,
gluteus maximus, hamstrings

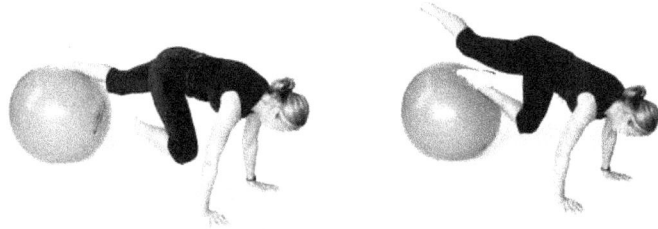

TWO BALL FROG KICK
PLANK POSITION
FEET ON BALLS

Primary muscles:
Iliopsoas, quads, gluteus
maximus, hamstrings,
transversus abd., multifidii

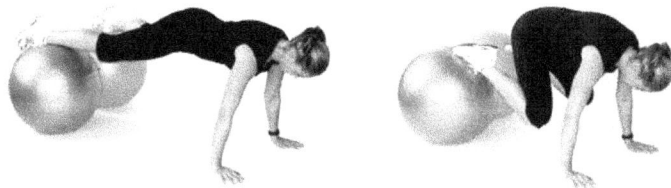

TWO BALL FROG KICK
ALTERNATING
PLANK POSITION

Primary muscles:
Iliopsoas, quadriceps,
gluteus maximus, hamstrings,
transversus abd., multifidii

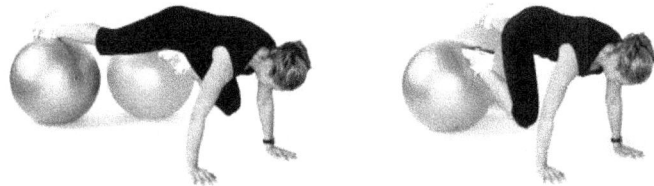

Plank position. Hands on the floor. Feet on the ball. Contract the abdominals and hip flexors and pull the knees and the ball towards the torso. Then contract the lower part of the abs to perform a pelvic tilt. Return. Press the legs into the ball to create resistance.	Core muscles stabilize. Neck in neutral position. Keep the buttocks low, in line with the rest of the body. This position may be hard on the wrists. The wrists should be strengthened gradually with few repetitions initially, short lever, more rest between sets.	Different arm position. With one or both legs.
Plank position. Hands on the floor. One lower leg on the ball, other leg free, off the ball, bent knee towards the torso. Pull in the leg and the ball towards the torso. Extend the free leg backwards. Repeat. After a set change leg.	Core muscles stabilize. Neck in neutral position. Keep the buttocks low, in line with the rest of the body. This position may be hard on the wrists. The wrists should be strengthened gradually with few repetitions initially, short lever, more rest between sets.	Different arm position.
Plank position. Two balls. One foot on each ball. Hands on the floor. Contract the hips and abs and pull the legs in towards the torso. Create resistance by pressing the legs into the ball. Extend the legs backwards.	Core muscles stabilize. Neck in neutral position. This position may be hard on the wrists. The wrists should be strengthened gradually with few repetitions initially, short lever, more rest between sets.	Different arm position.
Plank position. Two balls. One foot on each ball. Hands on the floor. Contract the hips and abs and pull one leg towards the torso. Extend the leg backwards. Change and pull the other leg in towards the torso and back out again.	Core muscles stabilize. Neck in neutral position. This position may be hard on the wrists. The wrists should be strengthened gradually with few repetitions initially, short lever and more rest between sets.	Different arm position. Perform the exercise with one leg at a time or alternate continuously.

**HIP EXTENSION
ONE BENT LEG
ON ALL FOURS ON THE FLOOR**

Primary muscles:
Transversus abdominis,
rotators, multifidii,
gluteus maximus, hamstrings

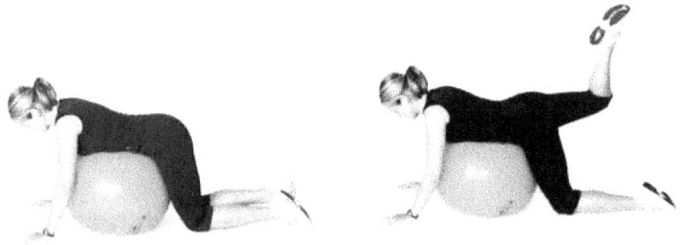

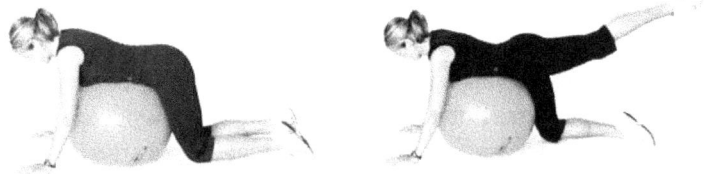

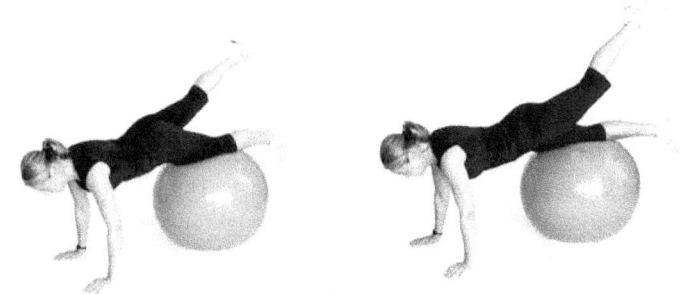

**HIP EXTENSION
ONE LEG (UNILATERAL)
ON ALL FOURS ON THE FLOOR**

Primary muscles:
Transversus abdominis,
rotators, multifidii,
gluteus maximus, hamstrings

**HIP EXTENSION
(PRONE HIP EXTENSION)
ONE LEG (UNILATERAL)
PRONE ON THE BALL**

Primary muscles:
Gluteus maximus, hamstrings,
transversus abd., multifidii

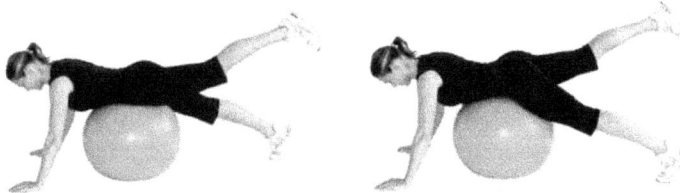

**HIP EXTENSION
ONE LEG (UNILATERAL)
PLANK, ONE LEG ON THE BALL**

Primary muscles:
Transversus abdominis,
rotators, multifidii,
gluteus maximus, hamstrings

On all fours on the ball. Ball under the abdomen. Hands on the floor. Bent legs. Lower legs on the floor. Lift one leg; thigh above horizontal. Lower. Repeat opposite. Legs remain bent throughout the exercise.	Good exercise for beginners. The stability ball should not be too big; you should lie comfortably across the stability ball. Core muscles stabilize. Neck in neutral position.	Different arm/leg position. Repeat or alternate.
On all fours on the ball. Ball under the abdomen. Hands on the floor. Bent legs. Lower legs on the floor. 1) Lift one leg; thigh above horizontal, 2) extend the knee, 3) flex the knee, 4) lower. Repeat or repeat with the opposite leg.	Combination exercise. The stability ball should not be too big; you should lie very comfortably across the stability ball. Core muscles stabilize. Neck in neutral position.	Different arm/leg position. Repeat or alternate.
Prone on the ball. Hands on the floor. Legs are straight, toes on the floor. Lift one leg above horizontal. Lower the leg. Repeat or repeat with the opposite leg.	Core muscles stabilize. Neck in neutral position.	Different arm/leg position.
Plank position. Hips or thighs on the ball. The legs are straight. Hands on the floor. Lift one leg, hip extension, approx. 10-15 degree angle to torso. Lower. Repeat or repeat with the opposite leg.	Stabilization exercise. Contract the core muscles to stabilize, keep the hips level and the body stable. Neck in neutral position. This position may be hard on the wrists. The wrists should be strengthened gradually with few repetitions initially, short lever, more rest between sets.	Different arm/leg position. Repeat or alternate.

**HIP EXTENSION
ONE LEG (UNILATERAL)
FOREARMS ON THE BALL**

Primary muscles:
Gluteus maximus, hamstrings,
transversus abdominis,
multifidii

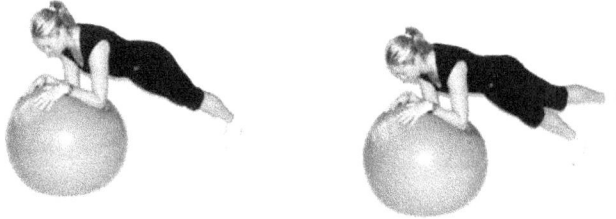

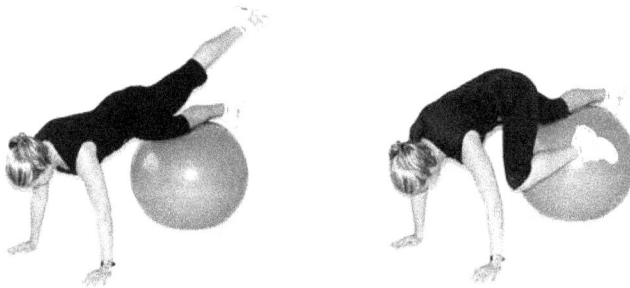

**HIP EXTENSION'N'FLEXION
UNILATERAL, PLANK
LOWER LEG ON THE BALL**

Primary muscles:
Gluteus maximus, hamstrings,
transversus abdominis,
multifidii

**HIP EXTENSION'N'FLEXION
SIDELYING ON THE BALL**

Primary muscles:
Transversus abdominis,
multifidii, rotators,
gluteus maximus, hamstrings,
iliopsoas, quadriceps

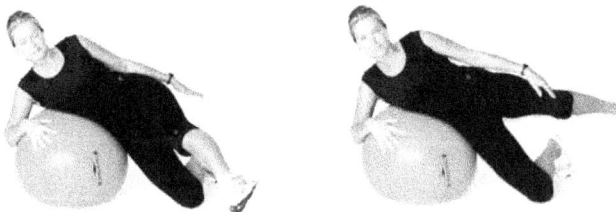

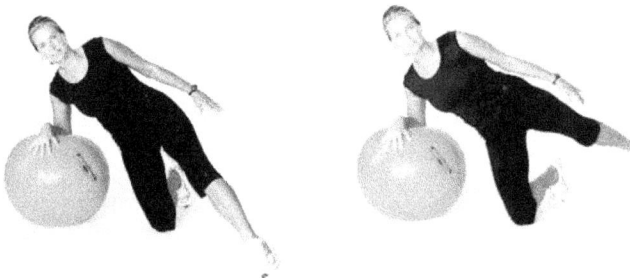

**HIP EXTENSION'N'FLEXION
SIDEPLANK POSITION**

Primary muscles:
Transversus abdominis,
multifidii, rotators,
gluteus maximus, hamstrings,
iliopsoas, quadriceps

Plank position. Hands or forearms on the ball. Legs are straight. Feet on the floor. Lift one leg; hip extension. Lower. Repeat or repeat with the opposite leg.	Contract the core muscles to stabilize. Neck in neutral position. For core and balance work.	Different arm/leg position.
Plank position. Hands on the floor. One thigh on the ball. The other leg, working leg, is lifted off the ball. Pull the leg in towards the torso. Extend the leg back into hip extension. Repeat with the same leg. After a set change leg.	Contract the core muscles to stabilize. Neck in neutral position. This position may be hard on the wrists. The wrists should be strengthened gradually with few repetitions initially, short lever, more rest between sets.	Different arm/leg position.
Sidelying on the ball. Bottom leg is bent, lower leg on the floor. Bottom arm around the ball. Top leg is straight and lifted into abduction. Move leg forward in front of the body and backward behind the body. Hip flexion and extension. Repeat. After a set change leg.	Stabilization and core exercise. Contract the core muscles to stabilize the body. Neck in neutral position.	Different arm/leg position.
Sideplank. Bottom leg is bent, kneeling on the lower leg by the side of the ball. Bottom forearm on the ball. Top leg is straight and lifted into abduction. Move leg forward in front of the body and backward behind the body. Repeat. After a set change leg.	For intermediate exercisers. Pilates type stabilizing exercise. Contract the core muscles to stabilize the body. Neck in neutral position.	Different arm/leg position.

**HAMSTRING PRESS
WITH BALL
PRONE ON THE FLOOR**

Primary muscles:
Hamstrings (Biceps femoris,
semitendinosus,
semimembranosus)

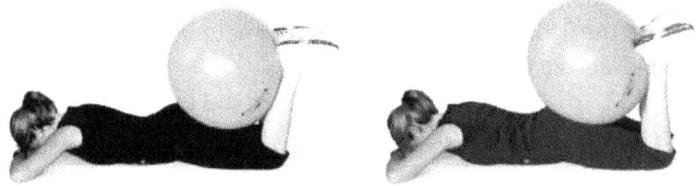

**HAMSTRING PRESS
ONE LEG (UNILATERAL)
SITTING ON THE BALL**

Primary muscles:
Hamstrings, transversus
abdominis, multifidii

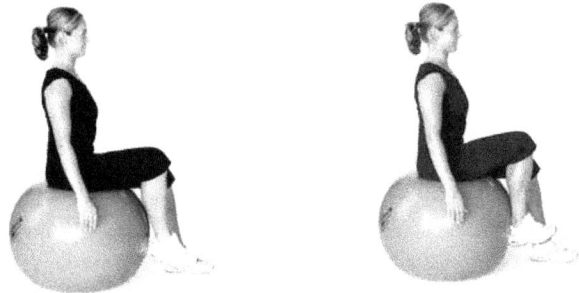

**HAMSTRING PRESS
WITH BALL
SUPINE ON THE FLOOR**

Primary muscles:
Hamstrings

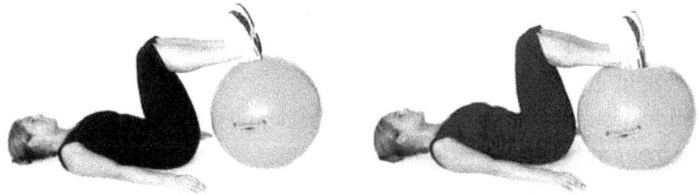

**HEEL MARCH,
BRIDGE POSITION
(OR SUPINE ON THE FLOOR)
HEELS ON THE BALL**

Primary muscles:
Gluteus maximus, hamstrings,
transversus abd., multifidii

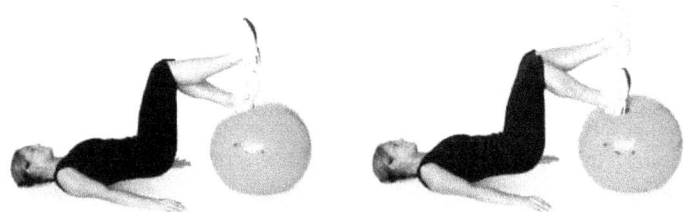

Prone on the floor. Hands under the forehead. The legs are bent and the ball is held tightly between the hamstrings and the heels. Bend the legs and press the heels deeper into the stability ball. Return with control.	Very small, almost isometric exercise. Limited functionality. To get into position: Start with torso upright, kneeling, with the ball resting on the lower legs, hold it, and go forward into prone position.	Different ballsize. One or both legs.
Sitting on the ball. The torso is erect. Arms down by the side. One foot on the floor. Other leg is lifted and bent. Press the heel into the stability ball. Release a little. Repeat. After a set change leg.	Very small, almost isometric exercise. Limited functionality. Contract the core muscles to stabilize.	Different arm position.
Supine on the floor. The arms are on the floor. The legs are bent. The heels are on the top of the ball. The hamstrings are close to the ball. Press the heels down into the stability ball. Release a little. Repeat.	Very Small, almost isometric exercise. Limited functionality.	With one or both legs. Dynamic, feet walking on top of the ball, heels press down into the stability ball.
Supine or bridge on the floor. The upper back and the arms are on the floor. The buttocks are contracted and the body is in bridge position. The legs are bent and perform a march on top of the stability ball with heels pressing into the ball.	Contract the core muscles to stabilize and keep the pelvis in neutral position.	Different arm position. **HAMSTRING PULL AND HAMSTRING STRETCH** Same exercise performed slowly. When one heel is pressed into the ball, the opposite leg is lifted vertically upwards or towards the torso.

PRONE KNEE EXTENSION
PLANK POSITION
LOWER LEGS ON THE BALL

Primary muscles:
Gluteus maximus, hamstrings,
quadriceps, iliopsoas, multifidii

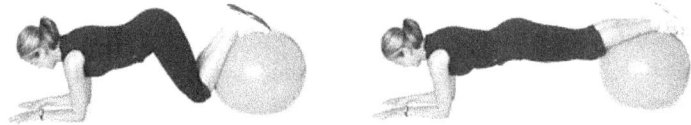

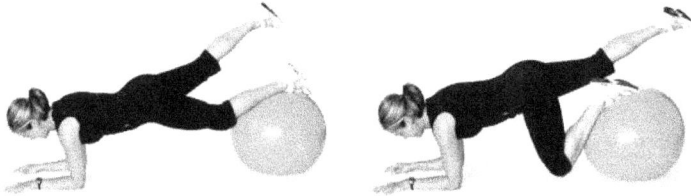

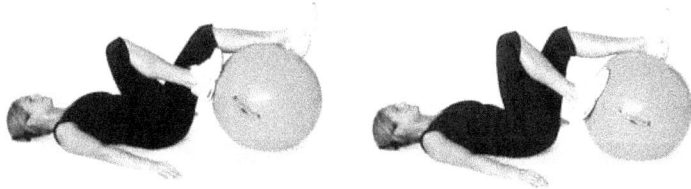

PRONE ONE-LEG
KNEE EXTENSION
PLANK POSITION
LOWER LEG ON THE BALL

Primary muscles:
Gluteus maximus, hamstrings,
quadriceps, iliopsoas, multifidii

HAMSTRING CURL AND
LEGPRESS
UNILATERAL
SUPINE ON THE FLOOR

Primary muscles:
Gluteus maximus, hamstrings,
quadriceps, iliopsoas

HAMSTRING BALL PULL
IN BALANCE
SITTING ON THE FLOOR

Primary muscles: Hamstrings,
rectus femoris, iliopsoas,
transversus abdominis,
multifidii, erector spinae

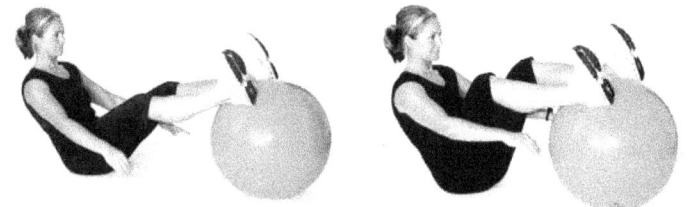

Plank position. Forearms on the floor. Lower legs on the ball. Press the lower legs into the ball. Bend the knees, stop when they are just above the floor. Extend the knees, while pressing the legs into the ball. Keep the body in a straight line, do not pike at the hips.	The ball should be fairly small. If it is not, then support yourself on the hands. Contract the core muscles to stabilize. Neck in neutral position.	Different arm/leg position. On forearms or hands. On both legs or one leg (for advanced exercisers).
Plank position. Forearms on the floor. One lower leg on the ball. Other leg is lifted off the ball. Bend the knee, stop when it is just above the floor. Extend the knee, while pressing down into the ball. Keep the body in a straight line, do not pike at the hips.	Contract the core muscles to stabilize. Neck in neutral position.	Different arm/leg position.
Supine on the floor. One lower leg on the ball with the heel pressed into the ball. The other leg is bent, the foot on the stability ball. The top leg tries to bend and pull the ball in, the bottom leg tries to extend and push the ball away from the body. Repeat opposite leg.	Isometric exercise. Limited functionality. Remember to keep breathing.	Different arm position.
Sitting on the floor. Arms down or forward. Legs are straight. The feet are on top of the ball or on each side of the ball. Contract the hamstrings and pull the ball towards the body. Extend the legs, return.	For intermediate exercisers. Requires some flexibility in the hamstrings. Contract the core muscles to stabilize. For core and balance work.	Legs hip-width apart, parallel, with heels on top of the ball, or legs apart, laterally rotated with the heels pressing into the side of the ball. Depending on leg position the effect changes slightly from hamstring to adductor focus.

**HAMSTRING CURL
WITH THE BALL
SUPINE ON THE FLOOR**

Primary muscles:
Hamstrings

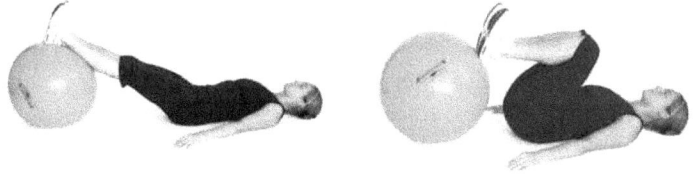

**HAMSTRING CURL
WITH THE BALL
BRIDGE, BACK ON FLOOR**

Primary muscles:
Gluteus maximus, hamstrings,
transversus abdominis,
multifidii

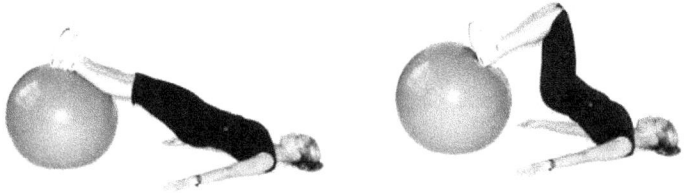

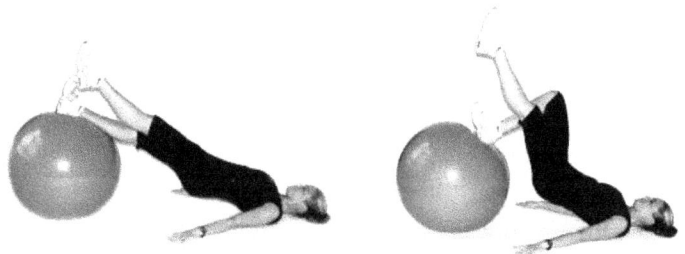

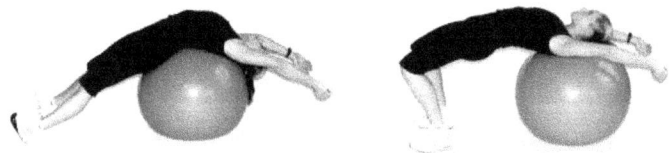

**ONE-LEG HAMSTRING CURL
WITH THE BALL
BRIDGE, BACK ON FLOOR**

Primary muscles:
Gluteus maximus, hamstrings,
transversus abdominis,
multifidii

**HAMSTRING CURL
SUPINE/BRIDGE ON THE BALL
HEELS ON THE FLOOR**

Primary muscles:
Gluteus maximus, hamstrings,
transversus abdominis,
multifidii

Supine on the floor. Arms on the floor. Legs straight, feet on the ball. The heels are pressing down into the stability ball. Bend the legs and pull the ball towards the buttocks. Extend the legs, return with control. Keep pressing the heels into the ball.	For beginners. Excellent hamstring exercise. The heels press into the ball at all times to create resistance. If all of the foot is in contact with the ball, adjust the position, so only the heels are pressing into the stability ball.	Different ballsize. One or both legs.
Bridge on the floor. The torso on the floor. Feet, heels, on the ball. The heels are pressing down into the stability ball. Bend the legs and pull the ball towards the buttocks. Extend the legs back out. Keep pressing the heels into the ball.	For beginning to intermediate exercisers. Excellent hamstring and buttock exercise. The heels press into the ball at all times to create resistance. If all of the foot is in contact with the ball, adjust the position, so only the heels are pressing into the ball.	Different arm position.
Bridge on the floor. Torso on the floor. One lower leg on the ball. The heel is pressing down into the stability ball. Bend the leg and pull the ball towards the buttocks. Extend the leg back out. Keep pressing into the ball.	Excellent hamstring and glute exercise. For intermediate exercisers. The heel presses into the ball at all times to create resistance. If all of the foot is in contact with the ball, adjust the position, so only the heel is pressing into the ball.	Different arm position. Different position of the free leg.
Supine across the ball. Lower back on the top of the ball. Arms out or back. Feet on the floor. Contract the hamstrings, bend the knees and pull the body forward to support on the upper back with the body in a bridge position. Return with control.	Contract the core muscles to stabilize. Keep the hips level. Press the torso down into the stability ball to increase resistance.	Different arm position.

**ABDUCTION
SIDELYING ON THE BALL**

Primary muscles:
Gluteus medius and minimus,
transversus abdominis,
multifidii

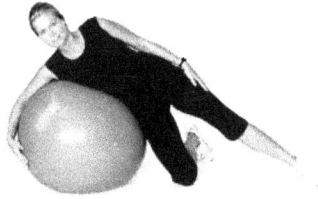

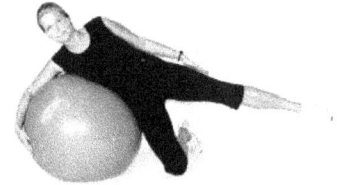

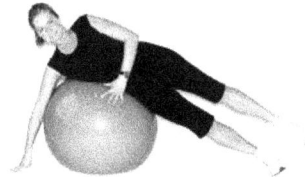

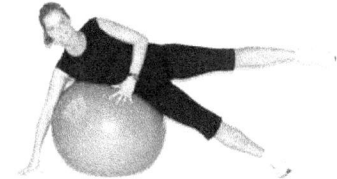

**ABDUCTION
SIDELYING ON THE BALL**

Primary muscles:
Gluteus medius and minimus,
transversus abdominis,
multifidii

**ABDUCTION
SIDEPLANK POSITION
ON THE BALL**

Primary muscles:
Gluteus medius and minimus,
transversus abdominis,
multifidii, quadratus lumborum

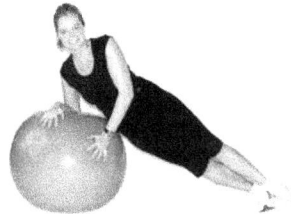

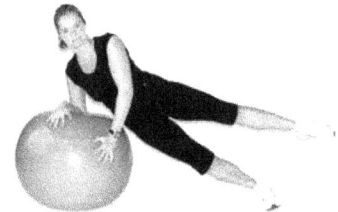

**ABDUCTION/ADDUCTION
SIDELYING ON THE FLOOR**

Primary muscles:
Gluteus medius and minimus,
adductors, transversus
abdominis, multifidii

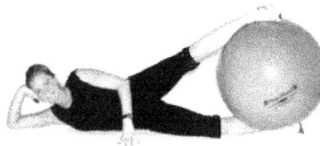

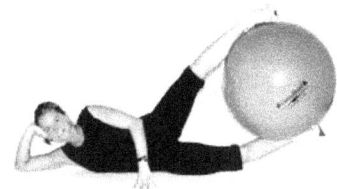

Sidelying on the stability ball. Top arm around the ball or by the side. Bottom arm hand is on the floor or around the ball. Inside leg is bent and lower leg is on the floor. Top leg is straight. Lift it up in the frontal plane, abduction. Lower. After a set change leg.	Core muscles stabilize. Neck in neutral position. Range of motion approx. 50 degrees abduction. Beyond that movement is caused by rotation at the hip or lateral flexion of the spine.	Different ballsize. Different leg position, straight or bent. Hip flexion will change the exercise: 45 degr.; tensor fascia latae, 90 degr.; gluteus maximus involvement.
Sidelying on the stability ball. Top arm around the ball or by the side. Bottom arm hand on the floor or around the ball. Both legs are straight, on top of one another or staggered. Lift the top leg up in the frontal plane, abduction. Lower. After a set change leg.	Core muscles stabilize. Neck in neutral position. Avoid lifting the head sideways. Range of motion approx. 50 degrees abduction. Beyond that movement is caused by rotation at the hip or lateral flexion of the spine.	Different arm position. Different leg position. **LEG CIRCLES** The top leg makes circles in the air. Change direction.
Sideplank position on the ball. The bottom arm is bent and the forearm is on the ball. The top hand is on the ball to stabilize the body and the ball. Both legs are straight, on top of one another or staggered. Lift the top leg up in the frontal plane, abduction. Lower. After a set change leg.	For advanced exercisers. Core muscles stabilize. Neck in neutral position. Avoid lifting the head sideways (as seen on the photo). Range of motion approx. 50 degrees abduction. Beyond that movement is caused by rotation at the hip or lateral flexion of the spine.	Different arm position free arm.
Sidelying on the floor. The arms are stabilizing the body. The stability ball is held firmly between the lower legs. Lift the legs up, sideways, in frontal plane. Lower.	Core muscles stabilize. Squeeze the ball to work the adductors effectively. The bottom arm may rest on the floor or support the head. Avoid lifting the head sideways away from neutral and do not push on the head with the hand.	Different arm position. The lower body and the ball can rotate forwards and backwards.

ADDUCTION
AND HAMSTRING PULL
SUPINE ON THE FLOOR

Primary muscles:
Gluteus maximus, hamstrings,
adductors

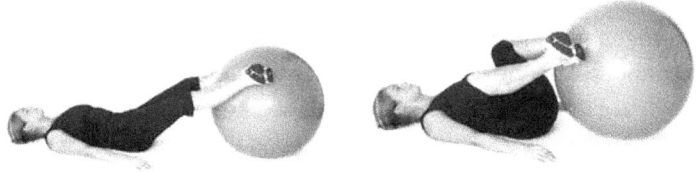

ADDUCTION
AND HAMSTRING PULL
BRIDGE POSITION
UPPER BACK ON THE FLOOR

Primary muscles: Gluteus
maximus, hamstrings,
adductors, erector spinae

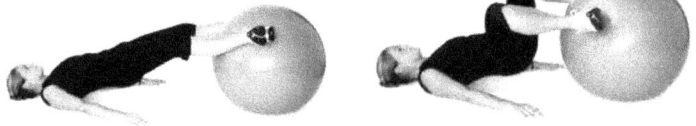

ADDUCTION
BALL BETWEEN THE LEGS
SUPINE ON THE FLOOR

Primary muscles:
Adductors

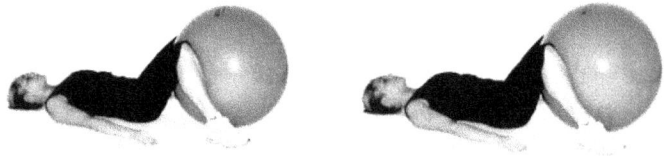

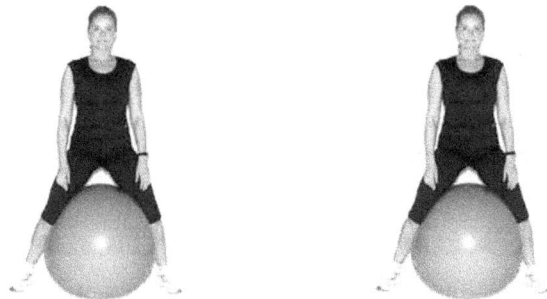

ADDUCTION
BALL BETWEEN THE LEGS
STANDING ON THE FLOOR

Primary muscles:
Adductors

Supine on the floor. Arms on the floor. Legs straight and apart. The heels press into the sides of the stability ball. Bend the legs and pull the ball towards the buttocks. Extend the legs with control.	Keep the legs rotated outwards throughout the exercise.

Keep pressing the heels into the ball to create resistance.

Contract the pelvic floor muscles when adducting the legs. | Different arm position.

Different ballsize. |
| Bridge on the floor. Upper back and arms on the floor. Legs straight and apart. The heels press into the sides of the stability ball. Bend the legs and pull the ball towards the buttocks. Extend the legs with control. | For intermediate exercisers.

Keep pressing the heels into the ball to create resistance.

Contract the pelvic floor muscles when adducting the legs. | Different arm position.

Different ballsize. |
| Supine on the floor. Arm position optional. Legs bent, feet on the floor. Stability ball between the legs. Adduct the legs and squeeze the ball. Release the pressure a little without relaxing. Repeat. | The stability ball shouldt not be too big.

Contract the pelvic floor muscles when adducting; do Kegel exercises at the same time. | Different arm position.

Different leg position. The feet can be on the floor or lifted; on the sides of the stabillity ball. |
| Standing on the floor. Arm position optional. The feet are apart; the stability ball is held between the legs. Adduct the legs and squeeze the ball. Release the pressure a little without relaxing. Repeat. | The stability ball should not be too big.

Contract the pelvic floor muscles when adducting; do Kegel exercises at the same time. | Different arm position. |

ADDUCTION
TOP LEG STRAIGHT
BOTTOM LEG BENT
SIDELYING ON THE FLOOR

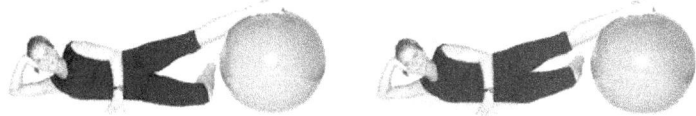

Primary muscles:
Adductors

ADDUCTION
WITH THE BALL
BETWEEN THE LEGS
SIDELYING ON THE FLOOR

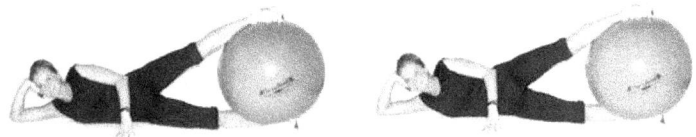

Primary muscles:
Adductors

ADDUCTION
SIDELYING ON THE BALL

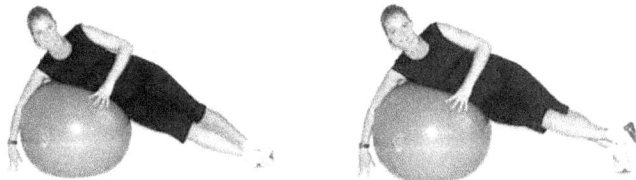

Primary muscles:
Adductors, multifidii,
transversus abdominis

ADDUCTION
SIDEPLANK POSITION
ARMS ON THE BALL

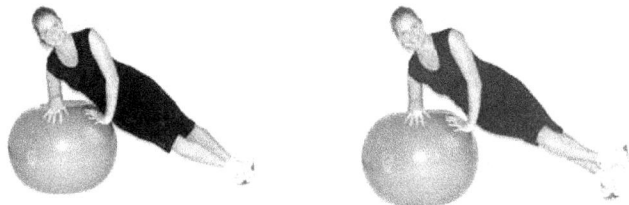

Primary muscles:
Adductors, multifidii,
transversus abdominis

146

Sidelying on the floor. Hips straight. The top leg is straight, the side of the foot is on top of the ball. The bottom leg is bent and on the floor. Lift, adduct, the bottom leg up into adduction. Lower the leg with control.	Contract the pelvic floor muscles when adducting the legs. The bottom arm can rest on the floor or support the head. Avoid lifting the head sideways away from neutral, and do not push on the head with the hand.	Different leg position. **ADDUCTION AND ROTATION** The bottom stays on the floor. The leg and knee rotate upwards towards the top leg.
Sidelying on the floor. Hips straight. The stability ball is held between the lower legs. Adduct the legs and squeeze the ball. Release the pressure a little without relaxing. Repeat.	Contract the pelvic floor muscles when adducting. The bottom arm may rest on the floor or support the head. Avoid lifting the head sideways away from neutral, and do not push on the head with the hand.	Different arm/body/leg position. You can lift the legs, in the frontal plane.
Sidelying on the ball. Bottom hand on the floor or arm around the ball. The legs are staggered; top leg is behind the bottom leg, foot on the floor to stabilize. Adduct and lift the bottom leg up into adduction, closely past the leg behind. Lower.	For lintermediate exercisers. Contract the core muscles to stabilize. Neck in neutral position. Avoid lifting head sideways. Contract the pelvic floor muscles when adducting.	Different arm/leg position.
Sideplank on the ball. The bottom arm is bent, forearm on the ball. Top arm forearm or hand on the ball. The body is on a straight line. Top foot on the floor behind the working leg. Adduct and lift the bottom leg, closely past the leg behind. Lower.	For advanced exercisers. Contract the core muscles to stabilize. Contract the pelvic floor muscles when adducting. Neck in neutral position. Avoid lifting the head sideways.	Different arm/body/leg position.

**HEEL LIFT (CALF RAISE)
SITTING ON THE BALL**

Primary muscles:
Soleus, gastrocnemeus

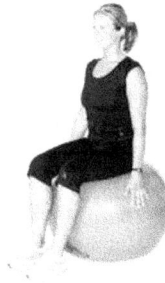

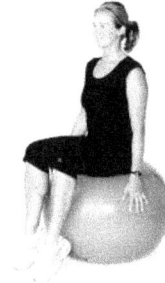

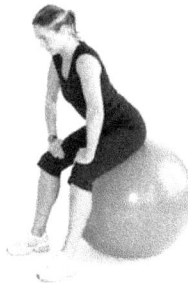

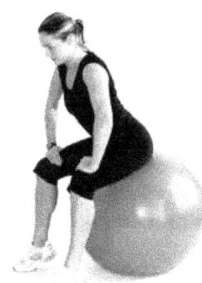

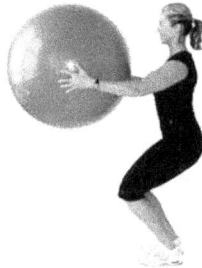

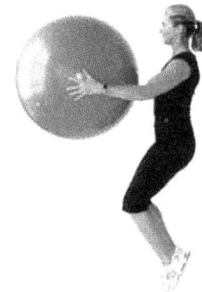

**HEEL LIFT (CALF RAISE)
WITH RESISTANCE
SITTING ON THE BALL**

Primary muscles:
Soleus, gastrocnemeus

**CALF RAISE, BENT LEGS,
STANDING ON THE FLOOR
WITH THE BALL IN HANDS**

Primary muscles:
Soleus, gastrocnemeus

**CALF RAISE,
STRAIGHT LEGS
STANDING ON THE FLOOR
WITH THE BALL IN HANDS**

Primary muscles:
Gastrocnemeus, soleus

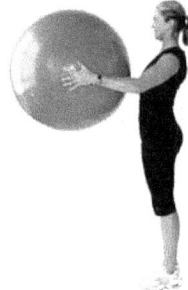

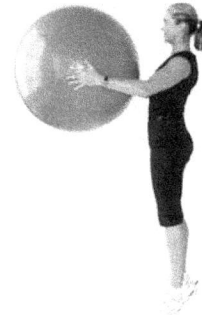

Sitting on the ball. The legs are bent, the feet are on the floor. The arms are down by the side. Contract the calf muscles and raise the heels as high as possible. Lower the heels with control.	Calf raise with bent legs, focus on the soleus. Leg work and very easy balance exercise.	With or without resistance. With both legs or one leg.
Sitting on the ball. The legs are bent, the feet are on the floor. The hands are on the thighs. Press the hands down on the thighs to create resistance. Contract the calf muscles and raise the heels; the thighs move up against the hands. Lower the heels with control.	Calf raise with bent legs, focus on the soleus.	With or without resistance. With both legs or one leg.
Standing on the floor. Feet together or shoulder-width apart on the floor. Legs bent. The ball is in the hands. The ball can be in front of the body or over the head. Raise the heels, lift up onto the toes. Lower the heels with control.	Calf raise med bent legs, focus on the soleus.	With or without resistance. Instead of the ball use a barbell or medicine ball. On both legs or one leg.
Standing on the floor. Feet together or shoulder-width apart on the floor. Legs straight. The ball is in the hands. The ball is in front of the body or over the head. Raise the heels, lift up onto the toes. Lower the heels with control.	Calf raise with straight legs, focus on the gastrocnemeus.	With or without resistance. Instead of the ball use a barbell or medicine ball. On both legs or one leg.

TOE RAISE (SHIN TAP)
SITTING ON THE BALL

Primary muscles:
Tibialis anterior

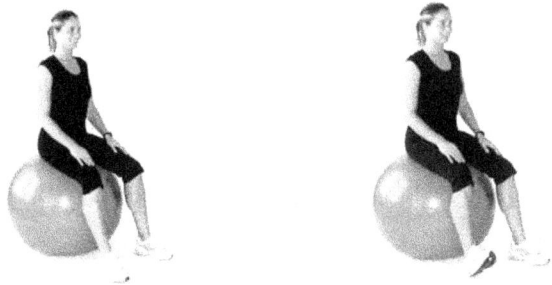

ANKLE FLEX'N'EXTEND
LOWER LEGS ON THE BALL
SUPINE ON THE FLOOR

Primary muscles:
Gastrocnemeus, soleus,
tibialis anterior

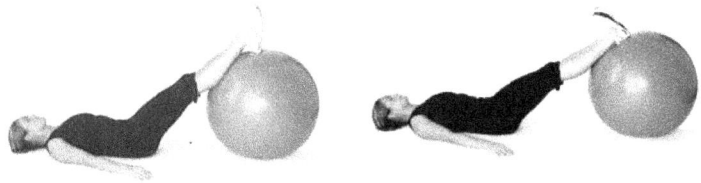

ANKLE-KNEE-HIP
FLEX'N'EXTEND
SUPINE ON THE FLOOR

Primary muscles: Tibialis
anterior, gastrocnemeus,
soleus, iliopsoas, hamstrings,
quadriceps, gluteus maximus

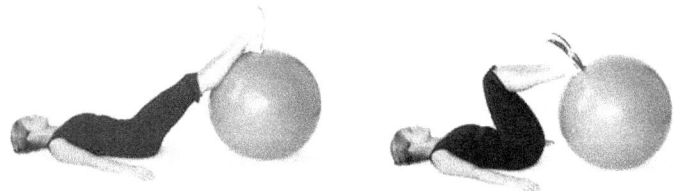

ANKLE-KNEE-HIP
FLEX'N'EXTEND,
BRIDGE ON THE FLOOR

Primary muscles: Hamstrings,
quadriceps, gluteus maximus,
gastrocnemeus, soleus,
tibialis anterior, iliopsoas

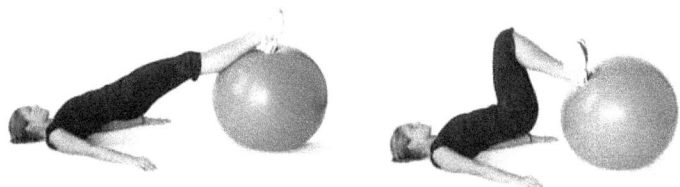

Sitting on the ball. Legs bent, feet on the floor. The arms are down by the side. Contract and pull the toes upwards towards the shins. Lower the toes with control.	The toe raise exercise is a supplement to your leg workout. For front lower leg activity.	With or without resistance: Support one end of a bodybar on the tip of the toes or have a rubber band over the toes and anchored below the stationary foot. With both legs or one leg.
Supine on the floor. Legs straight. Feet on top of the ball. Arms relaxed and on the floor. Flex and extend the ankles with control.	Very easy exercise for the lower legs. Increased mobility in the ankle, for increased range of motion, dorsiflexion, eg. for dancers and gymnasts.	Different arm/body/leg position.
Supine on the floor. Legs straight, lower legs on the ball. Bend the hips, the knees and the ankles and pull the ball towards the body. Extend the hips, the knees and the ankles and roll the ball back.	Easy exercise for the legs. Increased mobility in the ankle, for increased range of motion, dorsiflexion, eg. for dancers and gymnasts.	Different arm/body/leg position.
Bridge position on the floor. Legs straight, lower legs on the ball. Bend the hips, the knees and the ankles and pull the ball towards the body. Extend the hips, the knees and the ankles and roll the ball back.	Increased mobility in the ankle, for increased range of motion, dorsiflexion, eg. for dancers and gymnasts.	Different arm/body/leg position. With one or both legs.

8 | Ball And Equipment Exercises

In this section you find stability ball exercises for the major muscle groups in the upper and lower body and the torso, for one exerciser and one ball plus equipment such as rubberbands, bands, tubes, dumbbells, barbells and various stability training equipment.

The exercises are for intermediate to advanced exercisers.

The exercises are examples only, as there are numerous of other variations with different pieces of equipment.

Exercising with a ball and equipment requires a certain level of proficiency. You need some experience with stability ball training and resistance training as well as core strength in order to control the movements and stabilize the body.

Otherwise it will be too much at the same time, which will lead to a sloppy or faulty exercise technique, which results in a reduced workout effect or worse; injury, if you cannot control the ball and the equipment simultaneously. Please concentrate and progress with care.

In this section the ball is not used to create resistance, but works as a workout bench, which 1) facilitates a larger range of motion, than without the ball, 2) adds balance work and 3) works the core muscles along with the primary muscles of the exercise.

The exercises are listed by muscle groups and roughly 'from top to toe', not necessarily in the recommended sequence for a workout.

Most exercises can be varied by using one or both arms or legs and by changing the arm -, body - or leg position. All the exercises can be changed, made easier or harder, by using balls of different sizes and shapes and varying degree of inflation.

Important: All exercises are for healthy exercisers free from any serious or disabilitating disease, illness or ailments. Please consult your doctor before beginning these exercises.

Guidelines Elastic Resistance Training

Improve your elastic resistance training and avoid accidents by observing these precautions:

- Choose a suitable resistance. If you are unable to complete 8-12 repetitions, you should initially choose a lighter elastic band.
- Always check your equipment for wear and tear. Throw away broken bands and tubes. Elastic bands etc. should not be exposed to direct sunlight or water.
- Always check the joints between the elastic materials and the handles or straps.
- Always check that bindings and straps are firmly secured before starting the exercise.
- Elastic tubes – and bands – can be tied together and used as one piece of equipment, however, they are difficult to untie, so other alternatives are preferred.
- Do not wear rings, watches or jewellery when using elastic equipment.
- Do not press your fingers or nails into the elastic material.
- Do not maximally stretch a cold piece of elastic material to its maximum, warm it up a little, use exercises with a smaller range of motion.
- Do not stretch rubberbands and tubing over 2-3 times resting length.
- Do not stretch the resistance band over 3-5 times resting length (depending on brand).
- Always control the exercise, the pull of the elastic band, also during the eccentric phase.
- Protect you eyes. When you have checked the binding and exercise technique, look away from, do not look directly at, the elastic piece of equipment.
- The pull of the elastic piece of equipment should be in the direct opposite direction of the muscle (fibers) you wish to work.

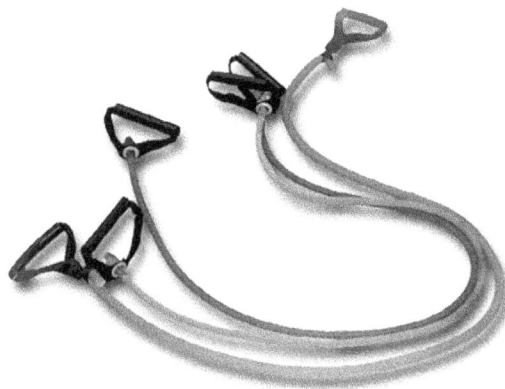

Guidelines Free Weight Resistance Training

Improve your free weight exercise program and avoid accidents by observing these simple precautions:

- Barbells and adjustable dumbbells: Equal load at both sides – and both dumbbells.
- Barbells and adjustable dumbbells: Secure the weight plates with a collar or clamp.
- Dumbbells in more parts: Check that the dumbbell is in one piece and the dumbbell weight plates are securely fastened.
- Barbells: Hold the bar with an even grip with both hands, so the bar is in balance.
- Barbells and dumbbells: Lift with a firm, closed grip, four fingers around the bar and the thumb closing. Do not use an *open* or *false grip* with all five fingers on one side, as you risk the weight falling from your hands onto your torso or limbs.
- Lift with proper lifting technique.
- Pay attention. Be careful not to accidentally drop barbells, dumbbells or weight plates.
- Put back the dumbbells in the rack, in pairs in their proper spot.
- Do not drop dumbbells or barbells, it is noisy and damages the dumbbells and flooring. Exception: When weightlifting in a weightlifting room with special flooring.

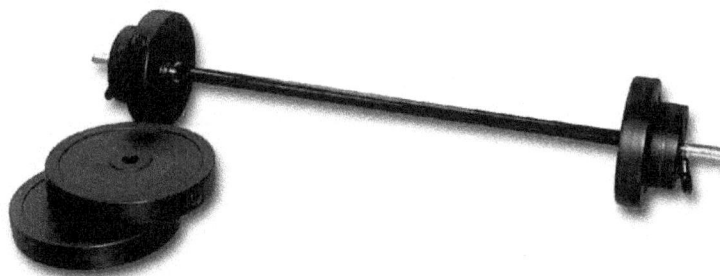

FRONT RAISE
WITH DUMBBELLS
SITTING ON THE BALL

Primary muscles:
Anterior deltoid

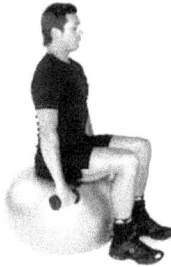

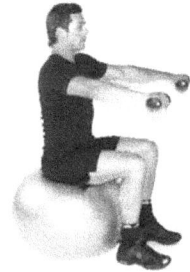

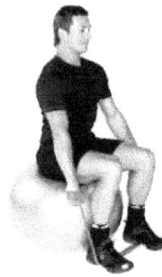

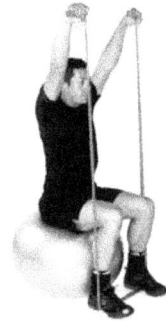

HIGH FRONT RAISE
WITH RESISTANCE BAND
SITTING ON THE BALL

Primary muscles:
Anterior deltoid

SHOULDER PRESS
WITH DUMBBELLS
SITTING ON THE BALL

Primary muscles:
Anterior and medial deltoid

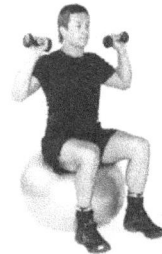

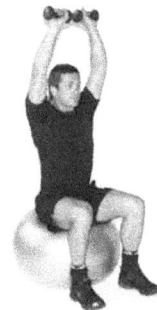

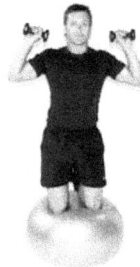

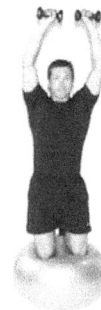

SHOULDER PRESS
WITH DUMBBELLS
KNEELING ON THE BALL

Primary muscles:
Anterior and medial deltoid

Sitting on the ball. Feet on the floor. A dumbbell in each hand. Arms at sides. Lift the arms forward and up to horizontal. Lower.	In this exercise there is a tendency to arch the lower back. Avoid this, contract the core muscles. Do not swing the arms, focus on the negative phase and lower the arms with control.	Different body/leg position. Standing, sitting, kneeling. With one or both arms – at the same time or alternating. Straight or bent arms. Over-, under-, neutral grip. With dumbbells, barbell, tube, band or medicine balll.
Sitting on the ball. Feet on the floor. Band under the feet. Hold the ends of the band with the hands. Arms at sides. Lift the arms forward and up above the head past horizontal. Lower.	In this exercise there is a tendency to arch the lower back. Avoid this, contract the core muscles. Turn the palms to face each other as this minimizes the risk of shoulder impingement.	Different body/leg position. Standing, sitting, kneeling. With one or both arms, at the same time or alternating. Straight or bent arms. Over-, under-, neutral grip. With dumbbells, barbell, tube, band or medicine ball.
Sitting on the ball. Feet on the floor. Arms are bent, hands by the shoulders. Press the dumbbells upwards. When the upper arms pass horizontal, the forearms should be vertical. Extend the arms. Lower, until the upper arms are at sides again.	Can be hard on the back and the shoulder (if flexibility is limited). Note: Past horizontal there is risk of shoulder impingement. Use a neutral grip; palms face each other. Note: Full range of motion: Upper arms start and finish by the side of the torso with the hands at shoulder level.	Different body/leg position. Overhand grip or neutral grip.
Kneeling on the ball. Arms are bent, hands by the shoulders. Press the dumbbells upwards. When the upper arms pass horizontal, the forearms should be vertical. Extend the arms. Lower, until the upper arms are at sides again.	Can be hard on the back and the shoulders (if flexibility is limited). Note: Past horizontal there is risk of shoulder impingement. Use a neutral grip; palms face each other. Note: Full range of motion: Upper arms start and finish at sides with the hands by the shoulders.	Different body/leg position. Over-, under- or neutral grip. With rotation.

**ARNOLD PRESS
SITTING ON THE BALL**

Primary muscles:
Anterior and medial deltoid

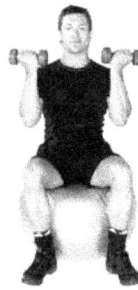

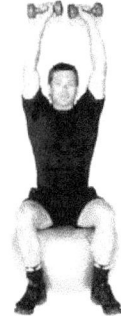

**UPRIGHT ROWING
WITH BARBELL
KNEELING ON THE BALL**

Primary muscles:
Anterior and medial deltoid,
biceps brachii

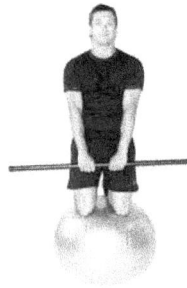

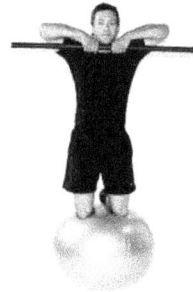

**AROUND THE WORLD
SUPINE ON THE BALL**

Primary muscles:
Deltoids, rotator cuff

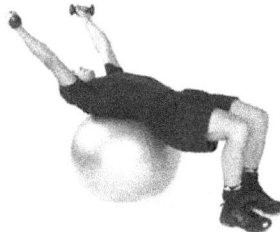

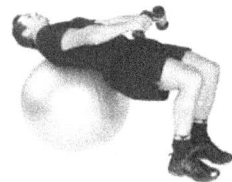

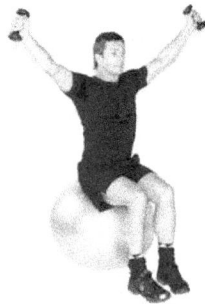

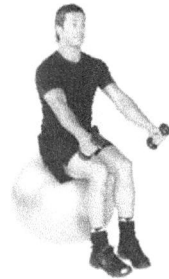

**AROUND THE WORLD
SITTING ON THE BALL**

Primary muscles:
Deltoids, rotator cuff

Sitting on the ball. Feet on the floor. Arms are bent and in front of the torso (as in biceps curl top position) with palms turned towards the torso. Dumbbells in hands. Press the arms up into vertical, shoulder press, while rotating the arms, so the palms turn forward away from the torso. Lower.	In top position the arms are rotated to a position, which may increase the risk of shoulder impingement. Alternative: Stop in neutral with palms facing each other. Extend the arms, but avoid hyperextending, locking, the elbows.	Different leg position. Standing, sitting, kneeling. With one or both arms – at the same time or alternating. With dumbbells, tube or band.
Kneeling on the ball. Narrow overhand grip on the barbell. Pull upwards, let the elbows lead, so they are slightly higher than the hands, which stop under the chin. Keep the wrists (close to) neutral. Lower with control.	Note: May cause shoulder impingement; stop when elbows are at or below shoulder level. When using a barbell, you find 'narrow grip' by grasping the middle of the barbell, putting the thumbs together, and then back around the barbell. They should not rest on the barbell.	Standing, sitting, kneeling. With one or both arms, at the same time or alternating. With dumbbells, tube or band. **UPRIGHT ROWING, WIDE** Wide overhand grip. The barbell is stopped at chest level (to reduce shoulder impingement).
Supine on the ball. Feet on the floor. Arms at sides, dumbbells in hands. The arms make a semi-circle (in the frontal plane, parallel to the floor) out and to a position 'overhead' (behind). Now the palms face each other. Raise the arms to vertical, then lower arms in front of the torso.	For stability, mobility and variety. Palms start facing the thighs, then they turn to face forward and in top position the palms face each other.	Different body/leg position. Prone. Sidelying with one arm.
Sitting on the ball. Feet on the floor. Arms at sides with dumbbells in hands. The arms make a semi-circle (frontal plane, parallel to the back wall) out and up overhead. Now the palms face each other. Lower the arms down in front of the torso.	For stability, mobility and variety. Palms start facing the thighs, then they turn to face forward and in top position the palms face each other.	Different body/leg position. Sitting, kneeling, standing on the ball.

**SIDE LATERAL RAISES, HIGH
WITH RESISTANCE BAND
SITTING ON THE BALL**

Primary muscles:
Anterior and medial deltoid

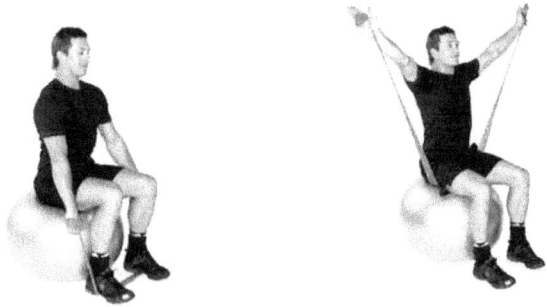

**SIDE LATERALS
(LATERAL RAISE)
WITH DUMBBELLS
SITTING ON THE BALL**

Primary muscles:
Medial deltoids

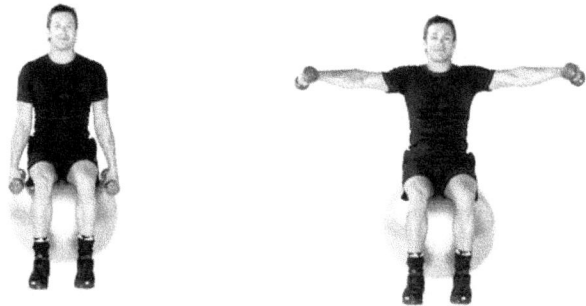

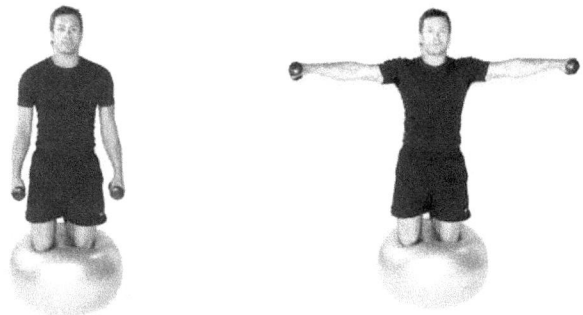

**SIDE LATERALS
WITH DUMBBELLS
KNEELING ON THE BALL**

Primary muscles:
Medial deltoids

**SIDE LATERALS, UNILATERAL,
WITH DUMBBELL,
SIDELYING ON THE BALL**

Primary muscles:
Deltoids, supraspinatus

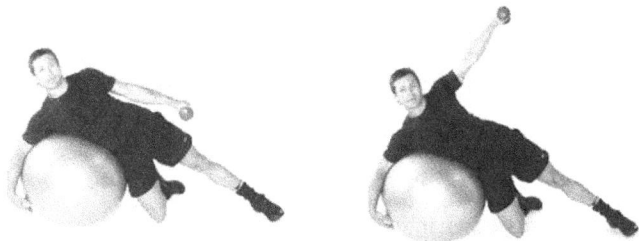

Sitting on the ball. Feet on the floor. Arms straight and at sides. The palms are facing the body, band around the hands. Lift the arms to the side and up above horizontal. The palms turn forward during the movement. Lower.	The arms are straight, but not hyperextended, the elbows are relaxed.	Different leg position. With one or both arms. Straight or bent arms.
Sitting on the ball. Feet on the floor. Arms straight and at sides. The palms are facing the body, dumbbells in the hands. Raise the arms to the side, to horizontal or a little below. Lower.	One of the main exercises for the medial deltoids. Raise the arms to a 60-80 degree angle only to reduce risk of shoulder impingement. Do not raise the arms above 90 degrees with the palms down. The arms, elbows, are straight, but not hyperextended.	Different leg position. With one or both arms.
Kneeling on the ball. Straight arms at sides. Arms straight, but not hyper-extended, elbows relaxed. The palms are facing the body, dumbbells in the hands. Lift the arms to the side, to horizontal or a little lower. Lower.	One of the main exercises for the medial deltoids. Raise the arms to a 60-80 degree angle only to reduce risk of shoulder impingement. Do not raise the arms above 90 degrees with the palms down. Above 80-90 degrees turn the palms forward or upward.	With one or both arms. Straight or bent arms.
Sidelying on the ball. Top arm straight and by the side, bottom arm around the ball. Top hand overhand grip on dumbbell. Raise the top arm to the side, perpendicular to the torso. Lower. Stop the movement just before the arm touches the leg. After a set repeat with the opposite arm.	The arm is straight, but not hyperextended, the elbow is relaxed.	Different body/leg position. The bottom arm supports on the floor or on the ball.

**SHOULDER FRONT RAISE
WITH DUMBBELLS
PRONE ON THE BALL**

Primary muscles:
Deltoids,
triceps brachii

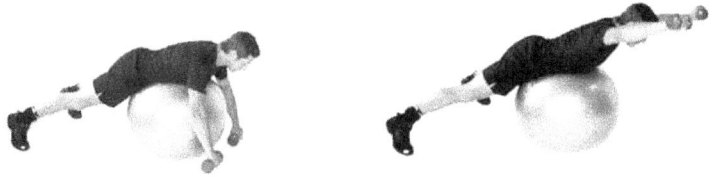

**SHOULDER EXTENSION
WITH DUMBBELLS
SITTING ON THE BALL**

Primary muscles:
Posterior deltoid,
triceps brachii

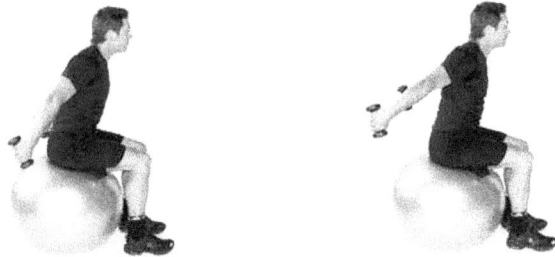

**BACK FLYE, UNILATERAL,
WITH DUMBBELL,
SIDELYING ON THE BALL**

Primary muscles:
Posterior deltoid

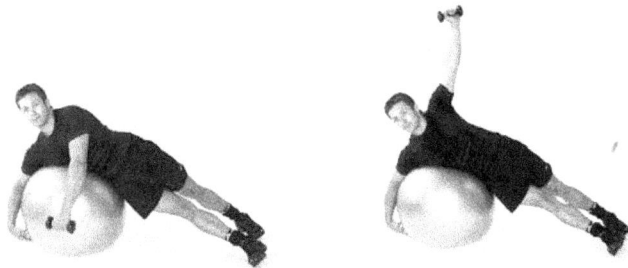

**UNILATERAL PULLOVER
WITH DUMBBELLS
BRIDGE ON THE BALL**

Primary muscles:
Deltoids, latissimus dorsi,
pectoralis minor

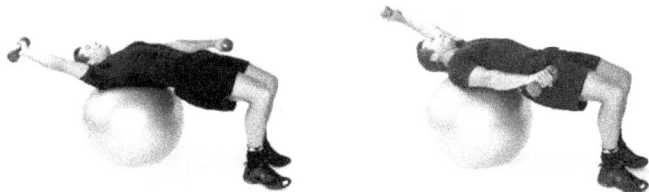

Prone on the ball. Toes on the floor. Arms straight and down in front of the ball. Dumbbells in hands. Lift the arms straight upwards, arms close by the head, in the sagittal plane. Lower. Stop just before the dumbbells touch the floor.	The arms are straight, but not hyperextended, the elbows are relaxed. Keep the body on a straigt line. Keep the neck in neutral position, do not drop the head down or look forward.	Different leg position. The arms at different angles to the torso. One or both arms. With or without resistance.
Sitting on the ball. Feet on the floor. Arms straight and extended behind the body. Dumbbells in hands. Lift the arms straight backwards and upwards, sagittal plane. Lower. Stop just before the dumbbells touch the ball.	The arms are straight, but not hyperextended, the elbows are relaxed. Contract the core muscles to stabilize. Keep the neck in neutral, the ears over the shoulders.	Different leg position. The arms at different angles to the torso. One or both arms. With or without resistance.
Sidelying on the ball. Feet staggered on the floor. Bottom arm around the ball. Top arm straight and down in front of the torso. Overhand grip on dumbbell. Lift the arm up close to vertical position (perpendicular to torso). Lower with control.	The arms are straight, but not hyperextended, the elbows are relaxed. Contract the core muscles to stabilize. Neck in neutral position.	Different body/leg position. The bottom arm supports on the floor or on the ball.
Bridge position. Upper back on the ball. Feet on the floor. One arm down by the side of the torso, the other overhead by the side of the head. Dumbbells in hands. The arms change place in a straight up and down movement in the sagittal plane. The arms stop around horizontal. Repeat.	Stabilizing shoulder exercise. Contract the core muscles to stabilize. Neck in neutral position.	Different body/leg position. Prone, sitting, kneeling or standing. Straight or bent arms. Overhand grip or neutral grip.

**SHOULDER EXTENSION
WITH RESISTANCE BAND
SITTING ON THE BALL**

Primary muscles:
Posterior deltoid,
triceps brachii

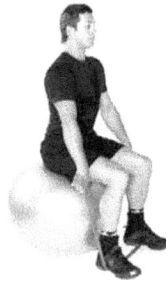

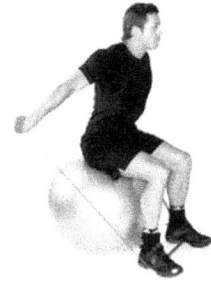

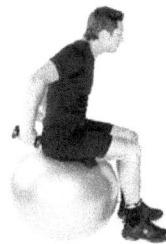

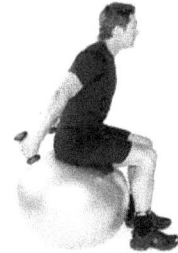

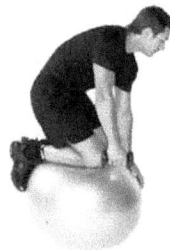

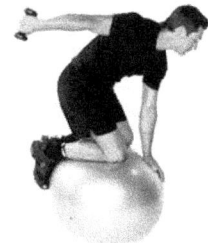

**SHOULDER EXTENSION
BENT ARMS
WITH DUMBBELLS
SITTING ON THE BALL**

Primary muscles:
Posterior deltoid,
triceps brachii

**SHOULDER EXTENSION
WITH DUMBBELLS
KNEELING ON THE BALL**

Primary muscles:
Deltoids, triceps brachii

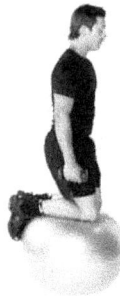

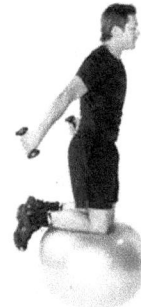

**SHOULDER EXTENSION
ONE ARM (UNILATERAL)
WITH DUMBBELL
ON ALL FOURS ON BALL**

Primary muscles:
Posterior deltoid,
triceps brachii

Sitting on the ball. Feet on the floor, band under the feet. Arms straight and at sides or just behind the torso. The hands hold the ends of the band. Lift the arms straight back, in the sagittal plane. Lower.	Neck in neutral position.	Different leg position. One or both arms. Bent or straight arms. Over-, under-, neutral grip. With dumbbells, barbell, tube or band.
Sitting on the ball. Feet on the floor. Arms straight and at sides or a little behind the torso. Dumbbells in hands. The arms straight back, in the sagittal plane. Arms bent. Lift and lower the arms (short lever shoulder extension).	Neck in neutral position.	Different leg position. One or both arms. Bent or straight arms. Over-, under-, neutral grip. With dumbbells, barbell, tube or band.
Kneeling on the ball. Arms straight and at sides (a little behind vertical). Dumbbells in the hands. Lift the arms straight back in the sagittal plane. Lift with the shoulders without moving the torso. Lower the arms. Stop before vertical position.	Contract the core muscles to stabilize. Neck in neutral position. Keep the arms/elbows straight.	Different arm/body position. With one or both arms. Straight or bent arms. Over-, under-, neutral grip. With dumbbells, barbell, tube, band.
On all fours on the ball. One hand on the ball. Lift the other arm, a dumbbell in the hand, straight back and up to or above horizontal. Lift with the shoulder without movement in the elbow or the torso. Lower. Stop before vertical position.	Contract the core muscles to stabilize. Neck in neutral position. Keep the arm/elbow straight.	Different arm/body position. Over-, under-, neutral grip.

**BACK FLYS
(PRONE REVERSE FLYS)
PRONE ON THE BALL**

Primary muscles:
Posterior deltoid,
rhomboids,
medial trapezius

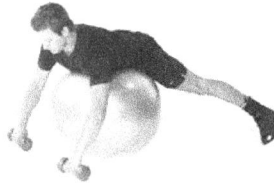

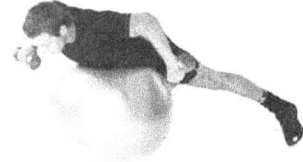

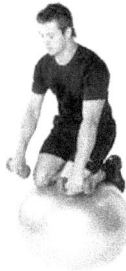

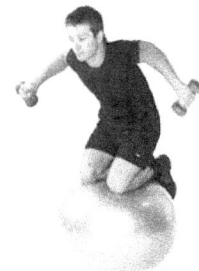

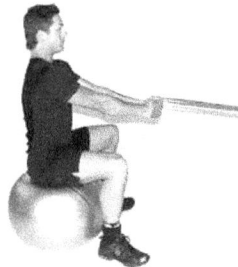

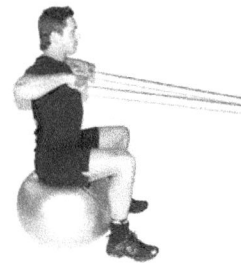

**BACK FLYS,
(REVERSE FLYS)
WITH DUMBBELLS
KNEELING ON THE BALL**

Primary muscles:
Posterior deltoid, rhomboids,
medial trapezius

**BACK FLYS, SITTING
(REVERSE FLYS)
WITH RESISTANCE BAND
SITTING ON THE BALL**

Primary muscles:
Posterior deltoid, rhomboids,
medial trapezius

**SHOULDER PRESS AND
BACK PULL
WITH RESISTANCE BAND
PRONE ON THE BALL**

Primary muscles:
Deltoids, latissimus dorsi,
trapezius

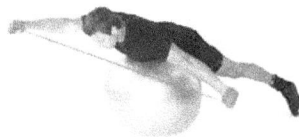

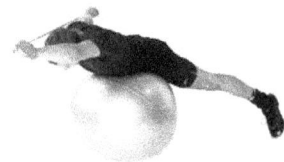

Prone. Toes on the floor. The arms are slightly bent and down in front of the body/ball. Dumbbells in the hands, overhand grip. Lift the arms to the side above horizontal. The elbows lead, and they remain slightly bent throughout the exercise. Lower.	Important postural exercise. First part of the exercise involves the back of the shoulders, last part of the exercise, when adducting the shoulder blades, involves the rhomboids and medial trapezius.	One or both arms. With or without resistance. On the floor, a ball or bench. **ARMS AT VARIOUS ANGLES** Overhead, 45° up and out, 45° down and out, and angles in between.
Kneeling on the ball. Torso slight forward lean. The arms are slightly bent and down in front of the body. Dumbbells in the hands. Lifts the arms to the side above horizontal plane. The elbows lead and remain slightly bent throughout the exercise exercise. Lower.	First part of the exercise involves the back of the shoulders, last part of the exercise, when adducting the shoulder blades, involves the rhomboids and medial trapezius. Be careful when leaning forward.	Different body/leg position. With or without support. Differet degree of hip flexion. One or both arms. With dumbbells, barbell, tube or band.
Sitting on the ball. Feet on the floor. Arms are slightly bent and forward in front of the body. The hands hold the ends of the band anchored in front of the body. Pull the arms out and back in horizontal plane. The elbows lead and remain slightly bent throughout the exercise. Return with control.	Important postural exercise. First part of the exercise involves the back of the shoulders, last part of the exercise, when adducting the shoulder blades, involves the rhomboids and medial trapezius.	Different leg position. One or both arms. Bent or straight arms. Overhand grip or neutral grip.
Prone on the ball. Toes on the floor. Band ind the hands. One arm is straight and lifted by the side of the head. The other arm is slightly bent and down by the side of the body. The arms change; back pull with almost straight arm and shoulderpress from bent to straight. Return with control.	Special exercise. For coordination and light resistance work.	Different leg position. Overhand grip or neutral grip.

**ROWING, WIDE, WITH
DUMBBELLS
(PRONE ROWING)
PRONE ON THE BALL**

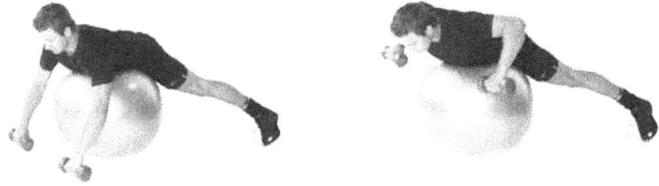

Primary muscles: Posterior
deltoid, rhomboids, medial
trapezius, biceps brachii

**BENT-OVER ROWING
ONE-ARM
WITH DUMBBELL
ON ALL FOURS ON BALL**

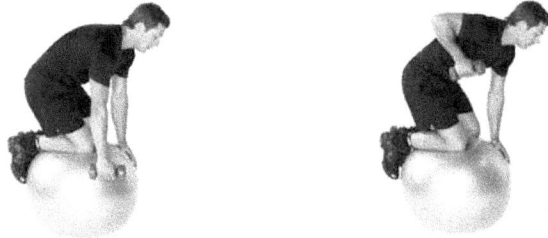

Primary muscles: Posterior
deltoid, rhomboids, medial
trapezius, biceps brachii

**ONE-ARM ROWING
WITH DUMBBELL
KNEELING ON THE BALL**

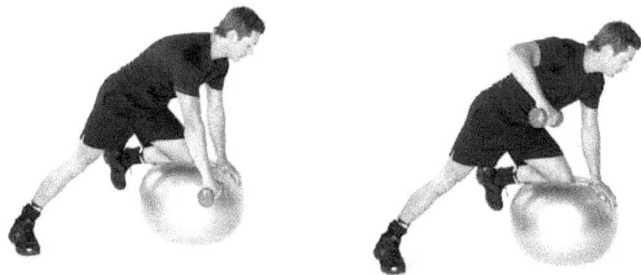

Primary muscles: Posterior
deltoid, rhomboids, medial
trapezius, biceps brachii

**ROWING, WIDE,
(SEATED ROWING)
WITH RESISTANCE BAND
SITTING ON THE BALL**

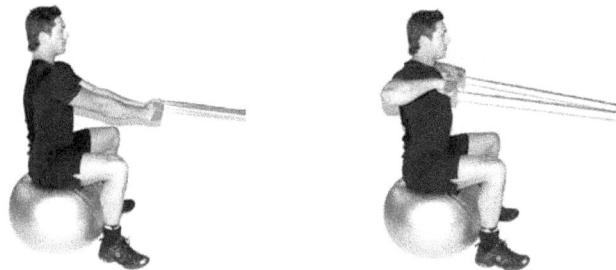

Primary muscles: Posterior
deltoid, rhomboids, medial
trapezius, biceps brachii

Prone on the ball. Toes on the floor. Arms down in in front of the ball and torso. Dumbbells in hands, overhand grip. Pull the arms up and back. In top position adduct the shoulder blades. Lower with control.	Important postural exercise. Use a high bench or a larger ball for a larger range of motion.	One or both arms. With or without resistance.
On all fours on the ball. One hand holds a dumbbell, overhand grip. Pull the arm up and to the side in a rowing movement. Upper arm above horizontal. Lower.	Important postural exercise. First part of the exercise involves the back of the shoulders, last part of the exercise, when adducting the shoulder blades, involves the rhomboids and medial trapezius.	Different body position.
Kneeling. One lower leg on the ball. Other foot on the floor. One hand (same side as the leg on the ball) on top of the ball. Torso leans forward. The other hand holds the dumbbell. Pull the arm ud and to the side. Upper arm above horizontal, Lower.	Important postural exercise. First part of the exercise involves the back of the shoulders, last part of the exercise, when adducting the shoulder blades, involves the rhomboids and medial trapezius.	Different body position.
Sitting on the ball. Feet on the floor. Arms straight and forward in front of the body. The hands hold the tube or band, which is anchored in front of the body. Pull the arms backwards in the horizontal plane, the elbows lead. Return with control.	Important postural exercise. First part of the exercise involves the back of the shoulders, last part of the exercise, when adducting the shoulder blades, involves the rhomboids and medial trapezius.	Different body position. With one or both arms.

SHOULDER UNILATERAL LATERAL ROTATION WITH DUMBBELL SIDELYING ON THE BALL

Primary muscles:
Infraspinatus

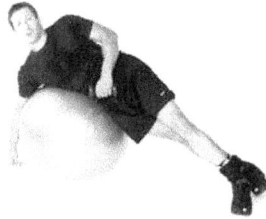

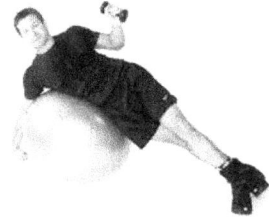

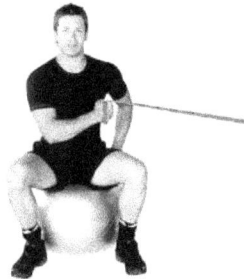

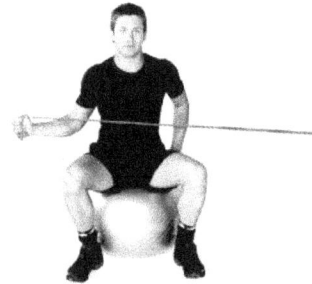

SHOULDER UNILATERAL LATERAL ROTATION WITH RESISTANCE BAND SITTING ON THE BALL

Primary muscles:
Infraspinatus

SHOULDER UNILATERAL MEDIAL ROTATION WITH DUMBBELL SIDELYING ON THE BALL

Primary muscles:
Subscapularis

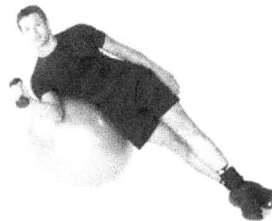

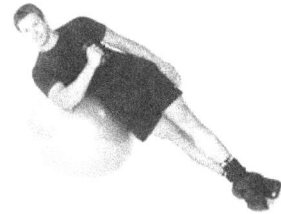

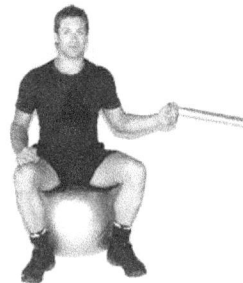

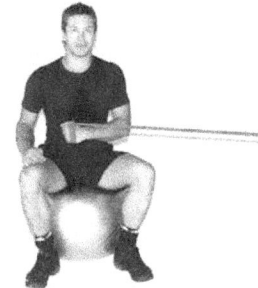

SHOULDER UNILATERAL MEDIAL ROTATION, WITH RESISTANCE BAND SITTING ON THE BALL

Primary muscles:
Subscapularis

Sidelying on the ball. Feet on the floor, staggered. Top upper arm close to the side, elbow bent 90 degrees. Elbow close to the hip. Keep the elbow in the same place throughout the exercise. Rotate the arm outward without the elbow moving.	Important shoulder stability exercise. The elbow should be close to the hip and stay in the same position throughout the exercise. The elbow should not slide back and forth, because this means, that the deltoid is taking over.	Different leg position. With or without resistance. Bottom hand on the floor or the stability ball.
Sitting on the ball. Feet on the floor. One upper arm close to the torso, elbow is bent 90 degrees, forearm in horizontal. Band is anchored by the side of the body at the opposite side. Hold the band with the hand. Rotate the arm outward without the elbow moving. Return with control.	Important shoulder stability exercise. The elbow should be close to the hip and stay in the same position throughout the exercise. The elbow should not slide back and forth, because this means, that the deltoid is taking over.	Different leg position. With rubberband, tube or band.
Sidelying on the ball. Feet on the floor, staggered. The bottom arm, elbow, is bent 90 degrees and close to the torso. Dumbbell in hand. The elbow is close to the hip. Rotate the arm inward, without the elbow moving. Return with control.	Important shoulder stability exercise. The elbow should be close to the hip and stay in the same position throughout the exercise. The elbow should not slide back and forth, because this means, that the deltoid is taking over.	Different leg position.
Sitting on the ball. Feet on the floor. Upper arm close to the torso, arm bent 90 degrees, forearm in horizontal. The hand holds the band. Rotate the arm inward without the elbow moving. Return with control.	Important shoulder stability exercise. The elbow should be close to the hip and stay in the same position throughout the exercise. The elbow should not slide back and forth, because this means, that the deltoid is taking over.	Different leg position. With rubberband, tube or band.

**CIRCLES ABOVE THE HEAD
WITH DUMBBELLS
SITTING ON THE BALL**

Primary muscles:
Deltoids, rotator cuff,
transversus abd., multifidii

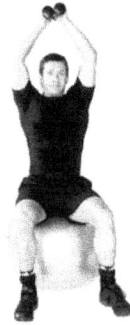

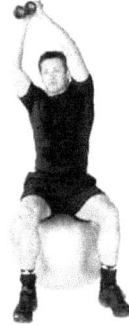

**REVERSE WOOD CHOP
WITH RESISTANCE BAND
SITTING ON THE BALL**

Primary muscles:
Posterior deltoid,
rhomboids, rotators

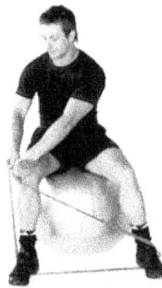

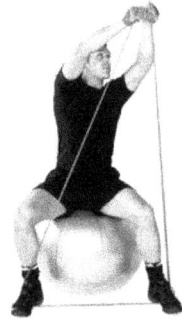

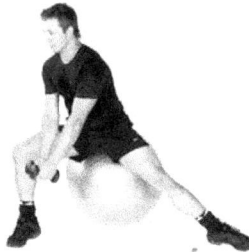

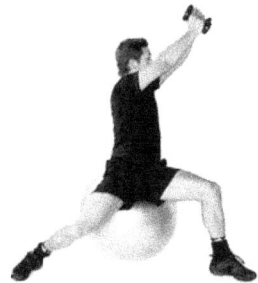

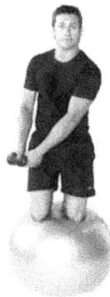

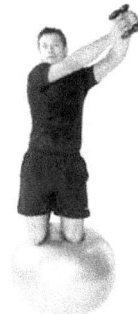

**REVERSE WOOD CHOP
WITH DUMBBELLS
SITTING ON THE BALL**

Primary muscles:
Posterior deltoid,
rhomboids, rotators

**REVERSE WOOD CHOP
WITH DUMBBELLS
KNEELING ON THE BALL**

Primary muscles:
Posterior deltoid,
rhomboids, rotators

Sitting on the ball. Feet wide apart on the floor. Both arms up above the head. dumbbell(s) in the hands. Move the arms in circles over the head. The core muscles contract to stabilize the body. Moderate tempo at the start. Repeat the opposite way.	Core exercise. Focus is on stabilizing the body, when the arms move.	Different arm/leg position. With dumbbells or a medicine ball.
Sitting on the ball. Feet wide apart on the floor. Hands in front of the body and to the side. The hands hold the ends of the band (anchored under the feet). Pull the arms and band diagonally upwards in front of the body to an overhead position at the opposite side. Lower.	Functional, compound exercise. After a set change side.	With one or both arms. With or without rotation. With tube or band.
Sitting on the ball. Feet wide apart on the floor. Arms down and together and to the side. Dumbbell(s) in hands. Lift the dumbbell(s) diagonally upwards to an overhead position at the opposite side. Lunge to the same side. Lower. Repeat. After a set change side.	For intermediate exercisers. Functional, compound exercise.	With one or both arms. With or without rotation. With or without lunge. With dumbbells or a medicine ball.
Kneeling on the ball. Arms down and together and to the side. Dumbbell(s) in the hands. Pull the arms diagonally upwards and in front of the body to an overhead position at the opposite side. Lower. After a set change side.	For advanced exercisers. Functional, compound exercise.	With one or both arms. With or without rotation. With dumbbells or a medicine ball.

**CHEST PRESS
WITH RESISTANCE BAND
SITTING ON THE BALL**

Primary muscles:
Pectoralis major,
anterior deltoid,
triceps brachii

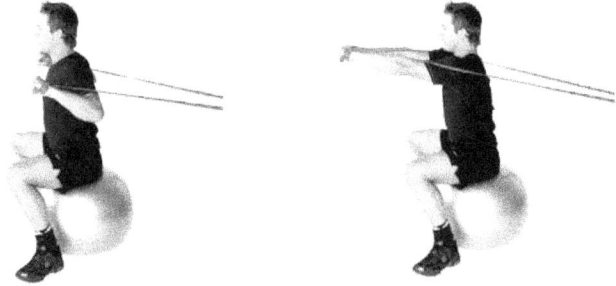

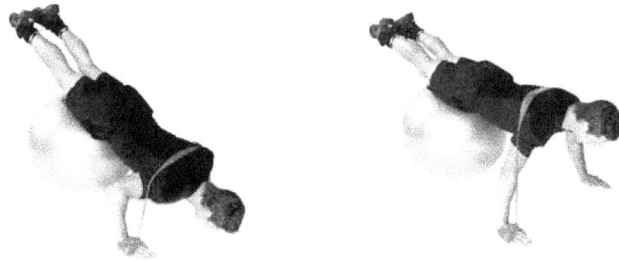

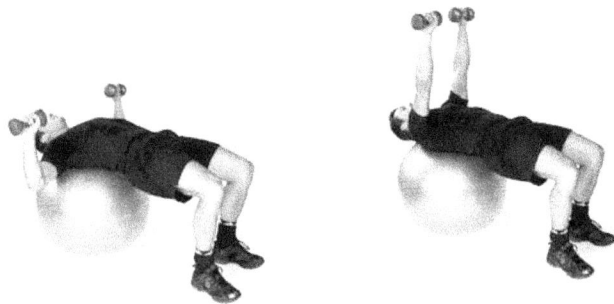

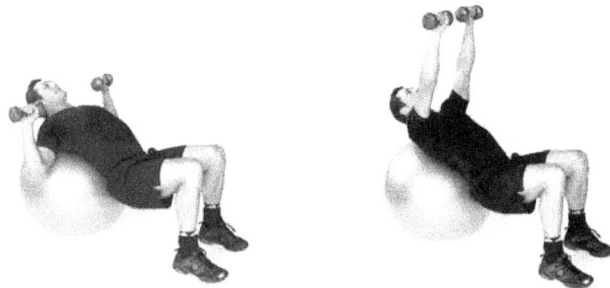

**PUSH-UP
WITH RESISTANCE BAND
PLANK POSITION
THIGHS ON THE BALL**

Primary muscles:
Pectoralis major, anterior
deltoid, triceps brachii

**CHEST PRESS
WITH DUMBBELLS
BRIDGE ON THE BALL**

Primary muscles:
Pectoralis major,
anterior deltoid,
triceps brachii

**INCLINE CHEST PRESS
WITH DUMBBELLS
SEMI-SUPINE ON THE BALL**

Primary muscles:
Pectoralis major, anterior
deltoid, triceps brachii

Sitting on the ball. Feet on the floor. Band anchored behind the body. Arms bent and to the side close to horizontal. The hands hold the ends of the band. Press the arms forward and together in front of the chest, Return with control. Stop when the upper arms are by the side of the torso.	Stop the return movement, when the upper arms are by the side of the torso. Do not let the arms move too far back as this hard on the shoulders.	Different arm/body/leg position. Different angle between the arms and the body.
Plank position on the ball. Legs together and lifted off the floor. Hands wide apart on the floor. Band around the upper back, the ends of the band anchored under the hands. The band is behind and under the arms. Bend the arms and extend the arms back up in a push-up.	Keep the band behind the arms and the shoulders or it will slip and roll up to the neck. (on photo 1, band has slipped off from behind the arms).	Different arm/leg position.
Bridge on the ball. Feet on the floor. Arms bent, upper arms to the side at shoulder level. Forearms vertical. Dumbbells in hands. Press the arms upwards into a vertical position above the chest. Lower with control. Stop when the upper arms are by the side of the torso.	Focus on the chest muscles. Stop the return movement, when the upper arms are by the side of the torso. Stop the upward movement just before vertical to keep working against gravity.	Different arm/body/leg position.
Semi-supine on the ball. Feet on the floor. Torso at an angle, incline position. Arms bent, upper arms to the side at shoulder level. Forearms vertical. Dumbbells in hands. Press the arms upwards into vertical position above the chest. Lower with control.	Stop the return movement, when the upper arms are by the side of the torso. Stop the upward movement just before vertical to keep working against gravity.	Different arm/body/leg position.

**CHEST FLYS
WITH DUMBBELLS
(SUPINE DUMBBELL FLYS)
BRIDGE ON THE BALL**

Primary muscles:
Pectoralis major, triceps
brachii, anterior deltoid

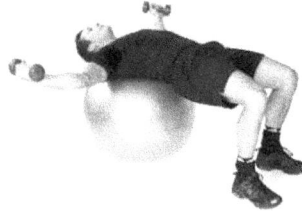

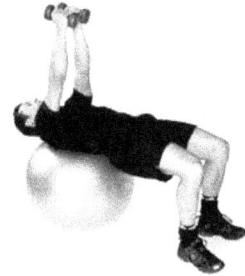

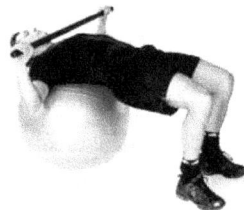

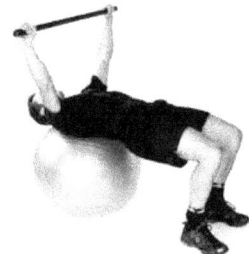

**INCLINE CHEST FLYS
WITH DUMBBELLS
(INCLINE DUMBBELL FLYS)
SEMI-SUPINE ON THE BALL**

Primary muscles:
Pectoralis major and minor,
triceps, anterior deltoid

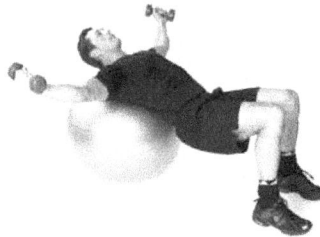

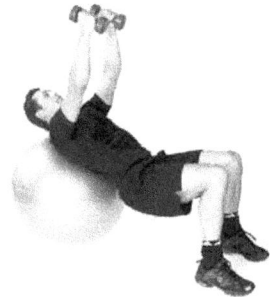

**BENCH PRESS
WITH BARBELL
(SUPINE BARBELL PRESS)
SUPINE ON THE BALL**

Primary muscles:
Pectoralis major, triceps
brachii, anterior deltoid

**STABILITY SHRUG
WITH DUMBBELLS
KNEELING ON THE BALL**

Primary muscles:
Trapezius, levator scapulae

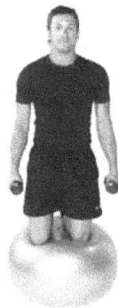

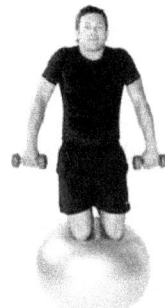

Bridge (or supine) on the ball. Feet on the floor. Arms slightly bent and to side in horizontal. Dumbbells in hands, palms face upwards. Lift the arms up and over the chest, stop just before vertical. Keep the elbow in the same position. Lower with control. Stop arms at shoulder level.	Stop the return movement, when the upper arms are by the side of the torso. Stop the upward movement just before vertical to keep working against gravity.	Different body/leg position. One or both arms. Different grip: Pronated, neutral grip (palms in), with rotation.
Supine on the ball. Feet on the floor. Torso in incline position. Arms slightly bent and to the side in horizontal. Dumbbells in hands, palms face upwards. Lift the arms up and over the chest, stop just before vertical. Keep the elbows slightly bent. Lower with control. Stop arms at shoulder level.	Stop the return movement, when the upper arms are by the side of the torso. Stop the upward movement just before vertical to keep working against gravity.	Different the bodys-/leg position. One or both arms. Different grip: Pronated, neutral grip (palms in), with rotation.
Bridge (or supine) on the ball. Feet on the floor. Hands hold barbell, wide grip. Wrists in neutral position. Barbell right above the forearms. Press the arms up, extend the elbows without hyperextending. Lower the barbell to the middle of the chest. Stop just before it touches the chest.	Stop the return movement, before the hands reach shoulder level, to reduce the load on the shoulder ligaments. Eg. stop approx ½ inch, 1 cm, above the chest. The arms can be angled slightly to further reduce the load on the shoulder ligaments.	With barbell or dumbbells. Different grip: Narrow grip (triceps focus) or wide grip (chest focus). **INCLINE BENCH PRESS** Perform in an incline position for more anterior deltoid work.
Kneeling on the ball. Arms at sides. Heavy dumbbells in the hands. Lift, shrug, the shoulders towards the ears. Lift in the frontal plane, do not pull the shoulders forward. Lower with control.	Assisting exercise for increased strength around the neck and shoulder girdle.	With dumbbells in both hands or in one hand only for increased core stability work. **CIRCULAR SHRUG** Pull the shoulders forward, up, backward and down. This does not increase the load (work) on the trapezius. It is a special exercise variation.

PULLOVER
WITH MEDICINE BALL
SUPINE ON THE BALL

Primary muscles:
Pectoralis major, serratus
anterior, latissimus dorsi

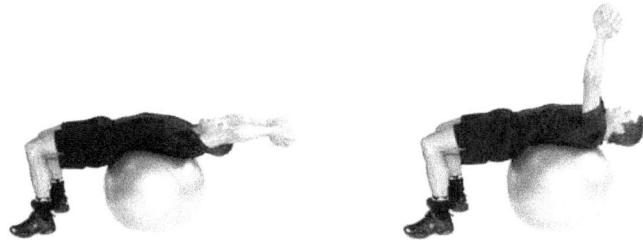

PULLOVER
WITH RESISTANCE BAND
SUPINE ON THE BALL

Primary muscles:
Latissimus dorsi, pectoralis
major, serratus anterior

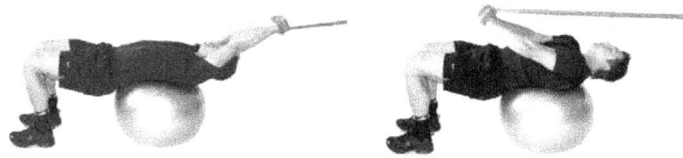

SEATED ROWING
WITH RESISTANCE BAND
NARROW GRIP
SITTING ON THE BALL

Primary muscles:
Latissimus dorsi, biceps brachii,
posterior deltoid

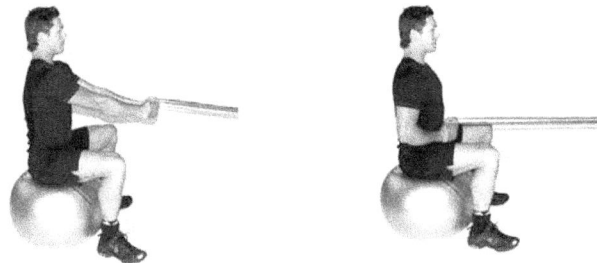

LAT PULL
WITH RESISTANCE BAND
PRONE ON THE BALL

Primary muscles:
Latissimus dorsi, biceps brachii

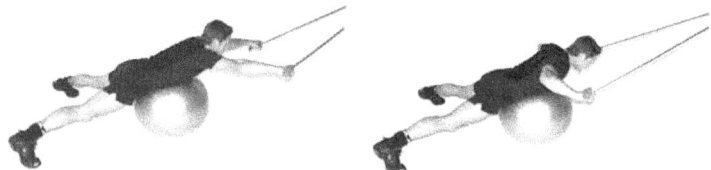

Supine on the ball. Feet on the floor. Arms vertical. Dumbbell or ball in hands. Lower the arms backwards behind the head. Stop the movement, when the upper arms are close to the ears. Pull the arms back up, stop just before vertical. The elbows remain straight throughout the exercise.	When using a dumbbell, use a triangle grip. Thumb and index finger of both hands around the dumbbell, touch each other and then slide them over one another to 'lock' the dumbbell in a firm grip. Stop upward movement just before vertical to keep working against gravity.	Different arm/body/leg position. Arms straight or slightly bent. With one or to dumbbells, barbell or medicine ball.
Supine on the ball. Feet on the floor. Band in the hands. Band anchored behind the body. Arms back, overhead, upper arms close by the ears. Pull the arms over the head forward and down over the torso. The elbows should remain straight throughout the exercise.	In pullover with a resistance band you work against resistance through a larger range of motion, than with dumbbells. Keep the arms straight, elbows straight, but not hyperextended, locked.	Different body/leg position.
Sitting on the ball. Torso erect. Feet on the floor. Tube/band anchored in front of the body. Arms forward in front of the torso. Pull the arms backwards, upper arms pass close by the side of the torso. Elbows lead. Keep the wrists in neutral. Return with control.	Contract the core muscles to stabilize.	Different body/leg position. One or both arms pull. Under-, over-, neutral grip. **ROWING, RHOMBOIDS** Arms to the side, in horizontal. Adduct the shoulder blades. **ROWING, LATISSIMUS DORSI** Arms close to the torso, pull elbows back behind the body.
Prone on the ball. Toes on the floor. Arms forward. Band anchored in front of the body. The hands hold the ends of the band. Pull the arms back and down, upper arms close to the side of the torso, in the frontal plane. Return with control.	Contract the core muscles to stabilize.	Different body/leg position. With tube or band.

**INCLINE BICEPS CURL
WITH DUMBBELLS
(BICEPS DUMBBELL CURL)
SEMI-SUPINE ON THE BALL**

Primary muscles:
Biceps brachii, brachialis,
brachioradialis

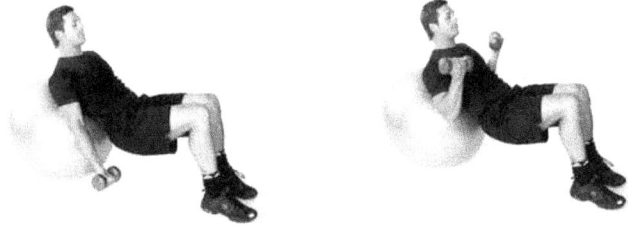

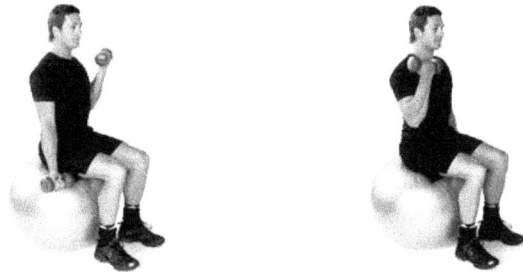

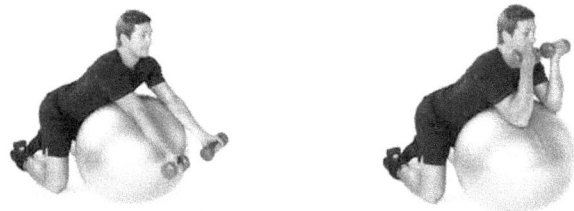

**BICEPS ALTERNATING
DUMBBELL CURL
SITTING ON THE BALL**

Primary muscles:
Biceps brachii, brachialis,
brachioradialis

**BICEPS BARBELL CURL
KNEELING ON THE BALL**

Primary muscles:
Biceps brachii, brachialis,
brachioradialis,
transversus abdominis,
multifidii

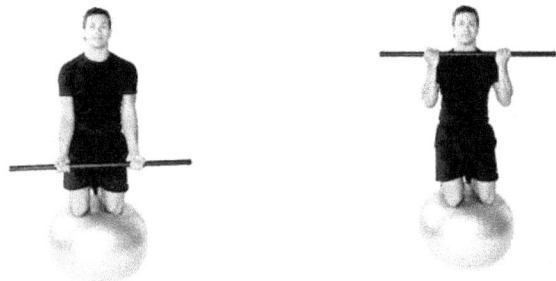

**BICEPS PREACHER CURL
ARMS ON THE BALL
KNEELING BEHIND THE BALL**

Primary muscles:
Biceps brachii, brachialis,
Brachioradialis

Semi-supine on the ball. Feet on the floor. The body in an incline position. Upper back against the ball. Arms down by the side, a dumbbell in each hand. Bend the arms, elbows. Elbows remain in the same position throughout the exercise. Lower with control.	Use full range of motion: 1) Bend the elbows almost completely, forearm close to vertical, but without losing tension. 2) Extend the arms completely, elbows extended, but not hyperextended.	Different body/leg position. Under, over- or neutral grip. With or without rotation. If using an overhand grip focus shifts from biceps to the brachialis and brachioradialis.
Sitting on the ball. Feet on the floor. Arms at sides, a dumbbell in each hand. Bend the arms alternatingly. Elbows remain in the same position throughout the exercise. Lower with control.	Alternate: One arm up and one down. Or let one arm complete the curl, before the opposite arm starts. One arm at a time makes it easier to isolate and focus, but keep contracting the arm, that is pausing. Tip: Start the movement from the top position, so the arm pausing is flexed, contracting.	Different body/leg position. Standing, sitting, kneeling. Under, over- or neutral grip. With or without rotation.
Kneeling on the ball. Contract the core muscles to stabilize the body. Arms down in front of the body. Hands shoulder-width apart holding a barbell, underhand grip. Bend the arms to lift the barbell. Elbows remain in the same place throughout the exercise. Lower with control.	Barbell curl is the number one isolation and mass exercise for the biceps brachii.	Different arm/body/leg position. Standing, kneeling. Under- or overhand grip.
Kneeling on the floor behind the ball. Lower legs on the floor. Torso on the ball. Upper arms on the ball. Hold dumbbell(s) with an underhand grip. Bend the arms to lift the dumbbells. Lower with control.	Isolation biceps work, with a somewhat limited range of motion.	Different body/leg position. Straight legs, body forward. With one or both arms.

**FRENCH PRESS, INCLINE
WITH DUMBBELLS
SEMI-SUPINE ON THE BALL**

Primary muscles:
Triceps brachii, deltoids

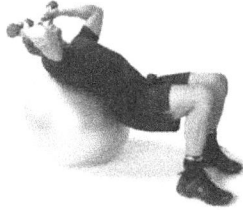

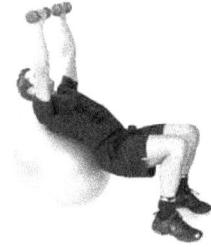

**FRENCH PRESS
WITH BARBELL
SUPINE ON THE BALL**

Primary muscles:
Triceps brachii, deltoids,
transversus abdominis,
multifidii

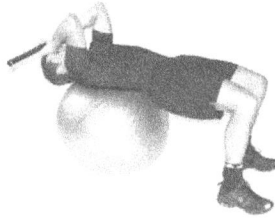

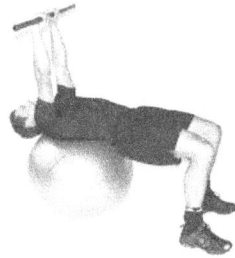

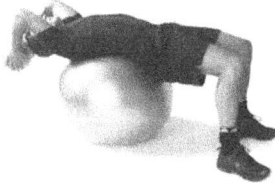

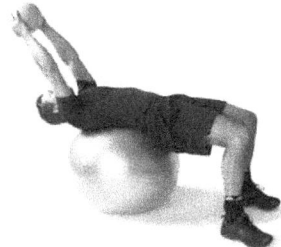

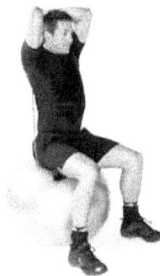

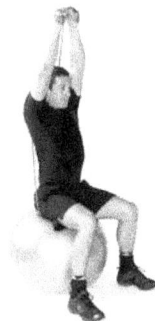

**FRENCH PRESS, 45 DEGR.
WITH MEDICINE BALL
SUPINE ON THE BALL**

Primary muscles:
Triceps brachii, deltoids,
transversus abdominis,
multifidii

**TRICEPS EXTENSION
WITH RESISTANCE BAND
SITTING ON THE BALL**

Primary muscles:
Triceps brachii, deltoids,
transversus abdominis,
multifidii

Supine on the ball. Feet on the floor. Torso in an incline position. Arms close to vertical. Dumbbells in hands. Bend the elbows, lower the hands and dumbbells close to the forehead or a little behind the head. Extend the arms, forearms up.	Use controlled movements. Use a spotter to check the technique. Keep the shoulders stable. Movement should be in the elbows.	Different leg position. Over-, under-, neutral grip. With dumbbells, barbell or medicine ball.
Supine on the ball. Feet on the floor. Barbell in the hands, shoulder-width apart. Arms close to vertical. Wrists neutral. Bend the arms, lower the barbell down just behind the forehead. Extend the arms, forearms up. Elbows should remain in the same place throughout the exercise.	Use controlled movements. Use a spotter to check the technique. Do not use the shoulders. Movement should be in the elbows. Keep the barbell in line with the forearm. Wrists neutral, do not 'drop' the wrists and the barbell backward.	Different leg position. With dumbbells, barbell or medicine ball.
Supine on the ball. Feet on the floor. The hands hold a medicine ball. The upper arms are backward, 45 degr. angle. Wrists in neutral. Bend the arms to lower the ball down behind the forehead, forearms vertical. Extend the arms back up. Elbows remain in the same place throughout the exercise.	Use controlled movements. Use a spotter to check the technique. Keep the shoulders stable. Movement should be in the elbows.	Different leg position. Over-, under-, neutral grip. On the floor, a bench or a ball. Flat, incline or decline bench. With dumbbells, barbell or medicine ball.
Sitting on the ball. Feet on the floor. Band anchored behind the body at a low position (or under the buttocks). The hands hold the ends of the band. The arms are overhead in vertical position. Bend the elbows and lower forearms with control. Extend the arms back up.	Contract the core to stabilize. Keep the upper arms vertical and shoulders stable. Movement should be in the elbows. Extend the elbows, but avoid hyperextionsion, locking. Elbows in the same position throughout the exercise.	Different leg position. Over-, under-, neutral grip.

**TRICEPS OVERHEAD
EXTENSION
WITH DUMBBELLS
KNEELING ON THE BALL**

Primary muscles:
Triceps brachii, deltoids,
transversus abd., multifidii

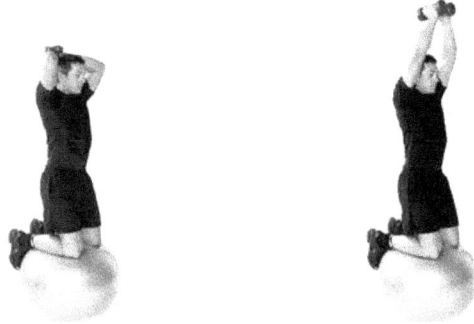

**TRICEPS KICK BACK
ONE-ARM WITH DUMBBELL
ON ALL FOURS ON THE BALL**

Primary muscles:
Triceps brachii,
posterior deltoid,
transversus abd., multifidii

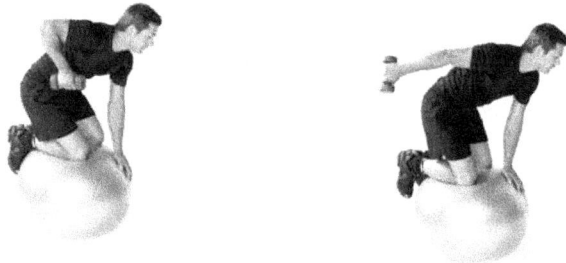

**BEHIND THE BACK
WRIST CURL
WITH BARBELL
SITTING ON THE BALL**

Primary muscles:
Wrist flexors

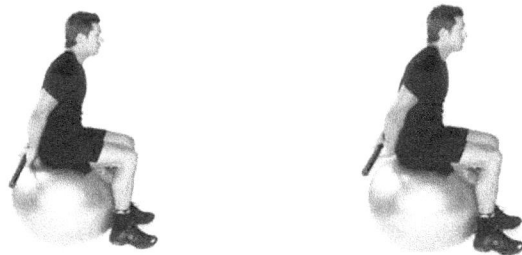

**REVERSE WRIST CURL
WITH DUMBBELLS
SITTING ON THE BALL**

Primary muscles:
Wrist extensors

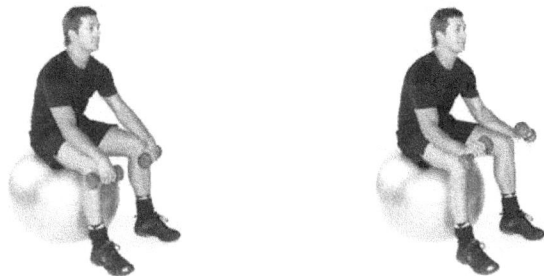

Kneeling on the ball. Contract the core muscles to stabilize. The upper arms are overhead. The hands hold the dumbbells. Bend the arms to lower the dumbbells with control. Extend the arms back up. Work in a full range of motion (elbows). The upper arms remain stationary.	Full range of motion: Full elbow flexion and extention (but no hyperextension).	With one or both arms.\n\nOver-, under-, neutral grip.
On all fours on the ball. Contract the core muscles to stabilize. One hand on the ball. The opposite hand holds the dumbbell. Upper arm in horizontal. Extend the elbow. Lower the forearm and dumbbell with control. Stop forearm just before vertical position.	Contract the core muscles to stabilize.\n\nUpper arm in horizontal, do not drop or swing it.\n\nWrist neutral, no movement. Movement should be in the elbow.	Different body position.\n\nOver-, under-, neutral grip.
Sitting on the ball. Feet on the floor. Barbell behind the body, in an underhand grip, palms face away from the body. Open the fingers and let the barbell roll down into the fingers. Bend the fingers and flex the wrists to roll the barbell up again.	Hold the barbell firmly. Avoid dropping it.	Different body/leg position. **FOREARM CURL** Sitting. Forearms on the legs. Underhand grip on barbell. Lower barbell by lowering the hands and opening the fingers, so the barbell rolls down in the fingers. Close the fingers again and flex the wrists as much as possible.
Sitting on the ball. Feet on the floor Forearms on the thighs. Wrists start in neutral position. Overhand grip on dumbbells. Lift the dumbbells by extending the wrist, lifting the hands back towards the forearms. Lower with control.	Hold the dumbbells with a firm grip, do not drop them on the toes.\n\nNote: For more training of the wrists and the fingers look for special literature on exercises with rubberbands, small balls or putty.	Different body/arm position.

**AB CURL
WITH BAND
SUPINE ON THE BALL**

Primary muscles:
Rectus abdominis, obliques,
transversus abdominis,
multifidii

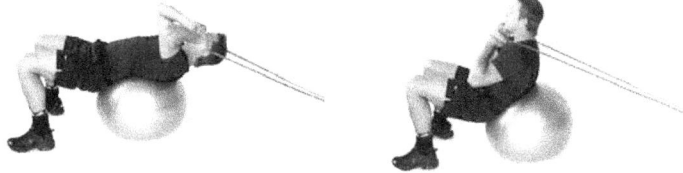

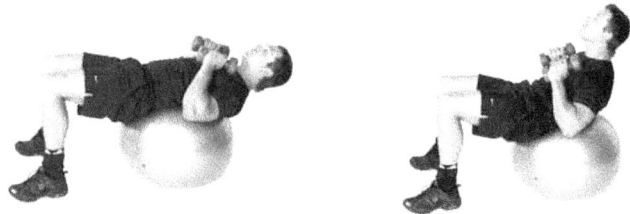

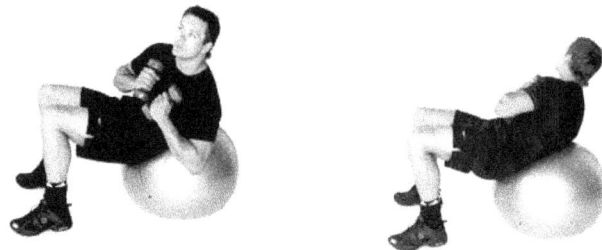

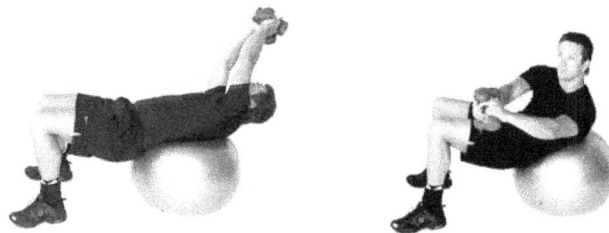

**AB CURL
WITH DUMBBELLS
SUPINE ON THE BALL**

Primary muscles:
Rectus abdominis, obliques,
transversus abdominis,
multifidii

**OBLIQUE CURL
WITH DUMBBELLS
SUPINE ON THE BALL**

Primary muscles:
Rectus abdominis, obliques,
transversus abdominis,
multifidii

**WOOD CHOP
WITH DUMBBELLS
SUPINE ON THE BALL**

Primary muscles:
Rectus abdominis, obliques,
transversus abdominis,
multifidii

Supine on the ball. Feet on the floor. Tube/band anchored behind the body. Ends of the band in the hands by the shoulders. Contract the abdominals and curl up the torso. Lower.	Contract the core muscles. Keep the neck in neutral position.	Different arm/body/leg position. With or without tube/band.
Supine on the ball. Feet on the floor. Dumbbell(s) in the hands by the shoulders or at the chest. Contract the abdominals and curl up the torso. Lower with control.	Contract the core muscles. Keep the neck in neutral position.	Different arm/body/leg position. With or without resistance. **PLATE CRUNCH** Ab curl with a weight plate (or dumbbell, medicine ball or barbell) held in straight arms in front of the chest.
Supine on the ball. Feet on the floor. Dumbbell(s) in the hands by the shoulders or at the chest. Contract the abdominals, curl up and rotate the torso. Rotate the shoulder towards the opposite hip. Lower. Repeat to the same or the opposite side.	Contract the core muscles. Keep the neck in neutral position.	Different arm/body/leg position. With or without resistance.
Supine on the ball. Feet on the floor. Arms diagonally up and over one shoulder. Both hands hold the dumbbell(s). Contract the abdominals, curl up and rotate towards the opposite hip. At the same time pull the arms diagonally across the torso towards the opposite thigh. Return. Repeat.	Contract the core muscles. Keep the neck in neutral position. Avoid 'throwing' movements with the arms and dumbbells. Use the obliques to move the torso, arms and dumbbells. After a set, repeat opposite.	Different arm/body/leg position.

**TORSO ROTATION
WITH TUBE/BAND
SITTING ON THE BALL**

Primary muscles:
Obliques internus and
externus, rotators, multifidii,
transversus abdominis

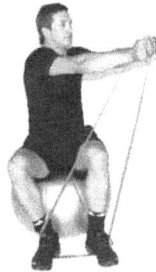

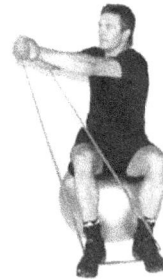

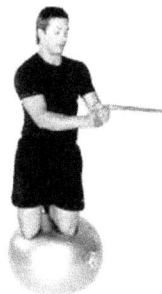

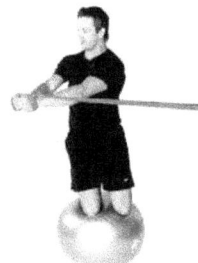

**TORSO ROTATION,
UNILATERAL
WITH TUBE/BAND
SITTING ON THE BALL**

Primary muscles: Obliques,
rotators, multifidii,
transversus abdominis

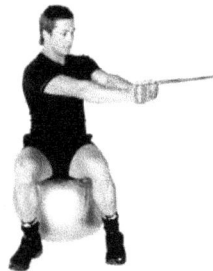

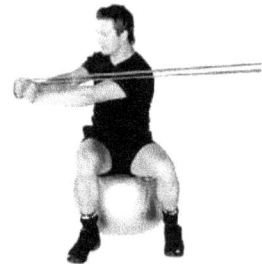

**TORSO ROTATION,
UNILATERAL, W. TUBE/BAND
KNEELING ON THE BALL**

Primary muscles:
Obliques internus and
externus, rotators, multifidii,
transversus abdominis

**TORSO ROTATION
WITH DUMBBELLS
KNEELING ON THE BALL**

Primary muscles:
Obliques internus and
externus, rotators, transversus
abdominis, multifidii

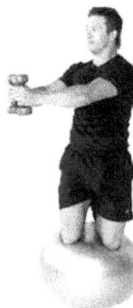

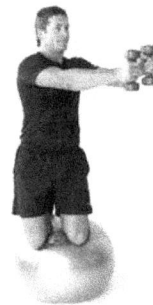

Sitting on the ball. Feet on the floor. Band under the feet. Hands together in front of the chest, ends of the band in the hands. Arms remain straight and in the same position throughout the exercise. Rotate the torso to one side. Return. Repeat other side.	Contract the core muscles to stabilize. Think of the spine as the axis of rotation. The head/neck rotates together with the spine to the side.	With tube or band.
Sitting on the ball. Feet on the floor. Tube/band anchored by a wall bar or a partner. Hold the ends of the band with the hands. Arms remain straight and in the same position throughout the exercise. Rotate the torso to the side. Return. Repeat. After a set change side.	Contract the core muscles to stabilize. Think of the spine as the axis of rotation. The head/neck rotates together with the spine to the side.	With tube or band.
Kneeling on the ball. Tube/band anchored by a wall bar or a partner. Hold the ends of the band with the hands. Arms remain straight and in the same position throughout the exercise. Rotate the torso to the side. Return. Repeat. After a set change side.	For advanced exercisers. Contract the core muscles to stabilize. Avoid moving the arms or legs. Think of the spine as the axis of rotation. The head/neck rotates together with the spine.	Different body position. Sitting, kneeling or standing on the ball. With tube or band. Rotate to one side at a time or alternate right and left.
Kneeling on the ball. Hold the dumbbell(s) with both hands. Arms straight and forward in front of the chest. Rotate the torso from side to side. Moderate tempo at the start.	For advanced exercisers. Contract the core muscles to stabilize. Avoid moving the arms or legs. Think of the spine as the axis of rotation. The head/neck rotates together with the spine.	Different body position. Sitting, kneeling or standing on the ball. With dumbbells or a medicine ball. In time increase the exercise tempo.

**SIDEBEND
WITH MEDICINE BALL
SIDELYING ON THE BALL**

Primary muscles:
Obliques internus and externus

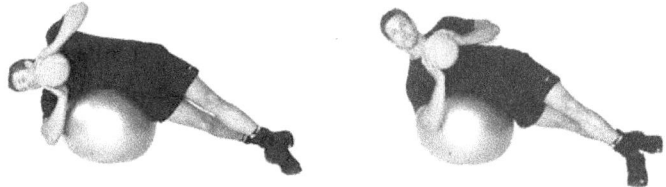

**SIDEBEND
WITH MEDICINE BALL
SIDELYING ON THE BALL
FEET ANCHORED**

Primary muscles:
Quadratus lumborum, obliques
internus and externus

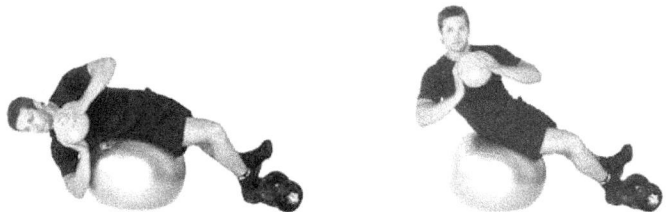

**BACK EXTENSION
WITH DUMBBELLS
PRONE ON THE BALL**

Primary muscles:
Erector spinae

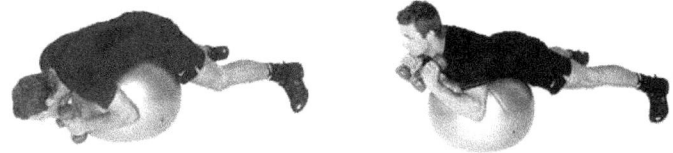

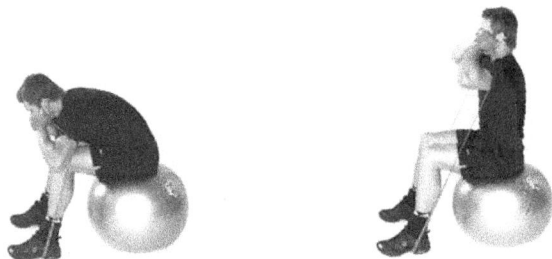

**BACK EXTENSION
WITH BAND
SITTING ON THE BALL**

Primary muscles:
Erector spinae

Sidelying on the ball. Legs are straight. Feet on the floor, staggered. Arms on the chest holding the medicine ball. Contract the obliques to sidebend the torso; shoulder straight towards same side hip. Lift as high as possible. Lower. After a set change side.	Contract the core muscles to stabilize. Lift the torso straight to the side. You can cross the lower legs with both feet sideways on the floor. Or stagger the feet on the floor, wide apart so the body is in a stable position.	Different arm position. Different leg position. With or without resistance.
Sidelying on the ball. Legs straight, feet anchored by a heavy dumbbell, wallbar or partner. Arms on the chest. The hands hold the medicine ball. Contract and sidebend the torso: shoulder straight towards same side hip. Lower. After a set change side.	Contract the core muscles to stabilize. Lift the body straight to the side. Important exercise for lower back stability. You can also use a BOSU or similar piece of equipment.	Different arm position. Different leg position. With or without resistance.
Prone on the ball. Toes on the floor, feet wide apart. Hands by the shoulders, holding the dumbbells. Contract the back extensors to lift the torso into back extension. Lower.	Contract the core muscles to stabilize. Neck in neutral position (on the right photo the head is lifted too much).	Different arm position. Back extension with rotation. Back extension with opposite arm/leg lift with dumbbells in the hands.
Sitting on the ball. Feet on the floor. Torso forward. Tube/band anchored under the feet. Hands by the side of the shoulders holding the ends of the band. Contract the back extensors and extend the torso up into upright position. Lower with control.	Contract the core muscles to stabilize. Keep the neck in neutral position.	Forskelllig arm/leg position. With band or tube. The band can also be anchored under the thighs.

**BALL WALL SQUAT
WITH DUMBBELLS
ON AN AEROSTEP**

Primary muscles:
Quadriceps, gluteus maximus,
transversus abd., multifidii

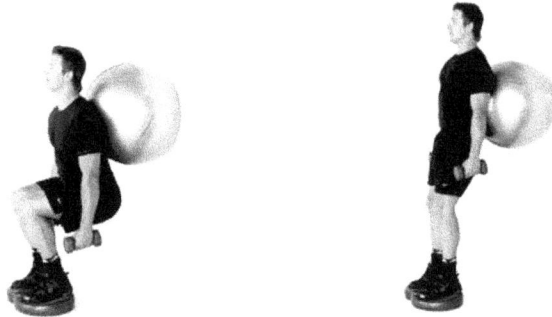

**ONE-LEG BALL WALL SQUAT
WITH DUMBBELLS
ON A STABILITY TRAINER**

Primary muscles:
Quadriceps, gluteus maximus,
hamstrings, TA, multifidii

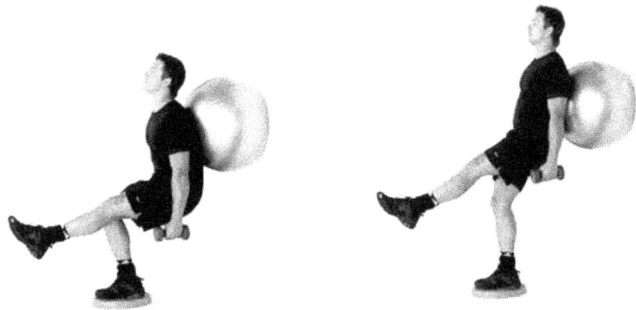

**SQUAT
WITH DUMBBELLS
STANDING ON THE BALL**

Primary muscles:
Quadriceps, gluteus maximus,
hamstrings, adductors,
transversus abd., multifidii

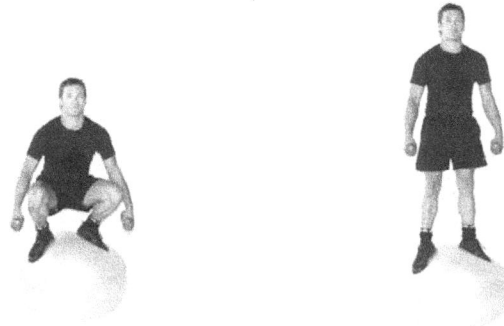

**DEADLIFT
WITH DUMBBELLS
KNEELING ON THE BALL**

Primary muscles:
Quadriceps, gluteus maximus,
hamstrings, erector spinae,
transversus abd., multifidii

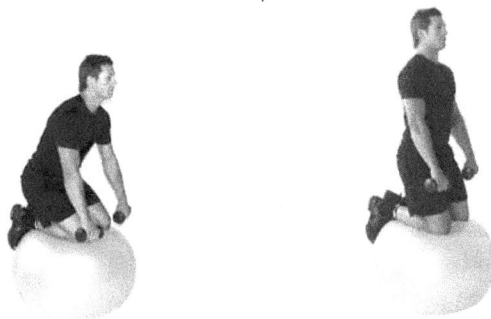

Standing on the floor. Feet on an aerostep. The back is on the ball, which is pressed against the wall. Dumbbells in hands. Bend the legs, squat down. Extend the legs. Return with control.	For beginning to intermediate exercisers. Be careful that the knees do not rotate inwards. Contract the thigh muscles and keep the knees aligned with the feet.	Different arm/leg position.
Standing on the floor. One foot on the stability trainer. Free leg straight and forward. The back is on the ball, which is pressed against the wall. Dumbbells in hands. Bend the leg, squat down. Extend the leg. Return with control.	For advanced exercisers. Contract the core muscles to stabilize. Be careful that the knee does not rotate inwards. Contract the thigh muscles and keep the knee aligned with the foot.	With or without resistance.
Standing on the ball. Arms at sides, dumbbells in hands. Torso erect, look straight forward. Feet firmly on the ball, approx. shoulder-width apart. Bend the legs, squat down. Extend the legs. Return with control.	For advanced exercisers. Note: High risk exercise. Contract the core muscles to stabilize. Be careful that the knees do not rotate inwards. Contract the thigh muscles and keep the knees aligned the feet.	With or without resistance.
Kneeling on the ball. Torso erect. Look straight forward. A dumbbell in each hand. Bend the hips and the knees, torso slightly forward, buttocks slightly back. Extend the hips and knees. Return to upright position with control.	For advanced exercisers.	Different body position. With or without resistance.

**LEG EXTENSION
WITH RUBBERBAND/BAND
SITTING ON THE BALL**

Primary muscles:
Quadriceps

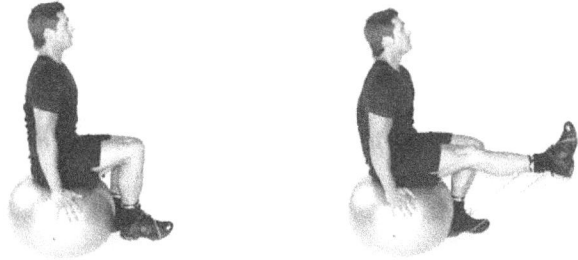

**LEG EXTENSION, ONE LEG
SITTING ON THE BALL
SUPPORTING FOOT
ON STABILITY DISC**

Primary muscles:
Quadriceps, transversus
abdominis, multifidii

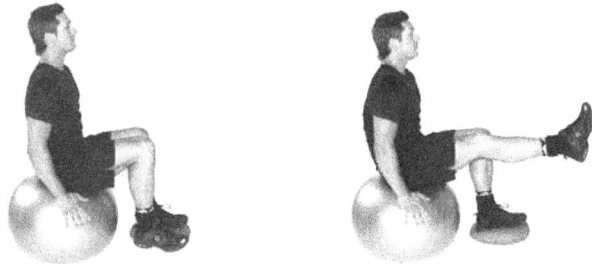

**HIP EXTENSION, ONE LEG
WITH RUBBERBAND/BAND
PRONE ON THE BALL**

Primary muscles:
Gluteus maximus, hamstrings

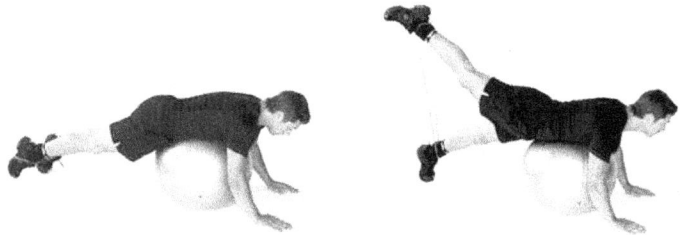

**HIP EXTENSION
(REVERSE HYPEREXTENSION)
PRONE ON THE BALL**

Primary muscles:
Gluteus maximus, hamstrings,
erector spinae

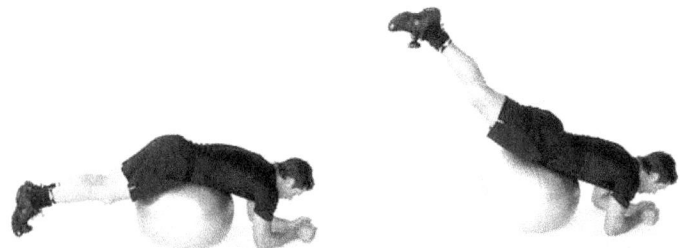

Sitting on the ball. Hands on the ball. One foot on the floor, other foot slightly lifted. Rubberband around both ankles or under the feet. Extend the knee of the lifted leg, lower leg to horizontal. Lower the lower leg with control.	Contract the core muscles to stabilize. Extend the knee complete with a controlled movement.	Different arm/leg position. With or without resistance.
Sitting on the ball. Hands on the ball. One foot on the floor on the stability disc. Other foot slightly lifted. Extend the knee of the lifted leg, lower leg to horizontal. Lower leg with control.	Contract the core muscles to stabilize. Extend the knee complete with a controlled movement. For quad and balance work.	With or without resistance.
Prone on the ball. Hands on the floor. Feet on the floor. Rubberband around both ankles. Hold one leg down, while lifting the other leg up into hip extension. Lower. Repeat with the same leg or the opposite leg.	Contract the core muscles.	With or without resistance.
Prone on the ball. Forearms or hands on the floor. Dumbbell held between the feet. Legs together. Contract the buttocks and the back extensors and lift the legs into hip extension. Lower with control.	Contract the core muscles to stabilize. If the dumbbell is heavy, it may be necessary to stabilize the body with the hands holding onto a wallbar.	Different body position.

LEG EXTENSION WITH BALL
PLANK, FEET ON THE BALL
HANDS ON A BOSU

Primary muscles: Quadriceps,
iliopsoas, gluteus maximus,
hamstrings, transversus
abdominis, multifidii

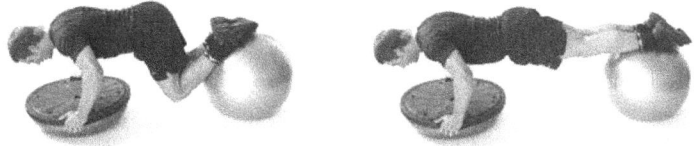

GOOD MORNING
WITH THE BALL
STANDING ON A BOSU

Primary muscles:
Hamstrings, gluteus maximus,
erector spinae, transversus
abdominis, multifidii

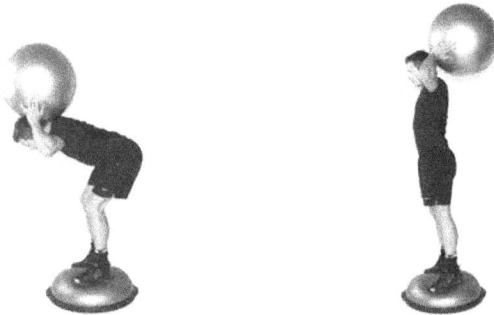

BULGARIAN SQUAT
BACK FOOT ON THE BALL
FRONT FOOT ON A
STABILITY TRAINER

Primary muscles: Quadriceps,
gluteus maximus, hamstrings,
multifidii, transversus abd.

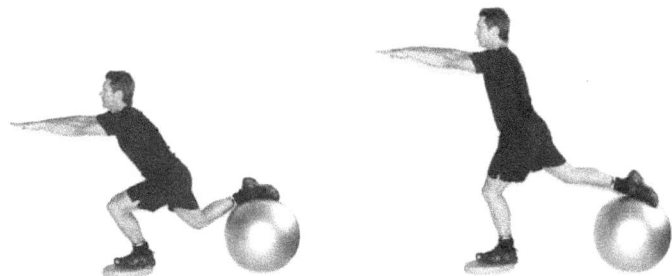

ONE-LEG LEG PRESS
RUBBERBAND/TUBE/BAND
ON ALL FOURS
TORSO ON THE BALL

Primary muscles:
Gluteus maximus, hamstrings,
quadriceps

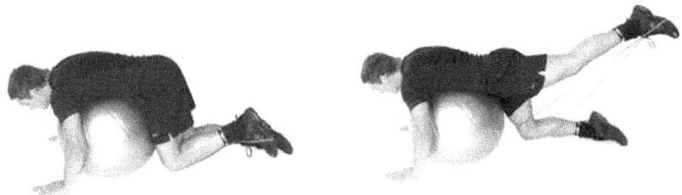

Plank position. Contract the core muscles to keep the body stable and on a straight line. Hands on a BOSU upside down. Lower legs on top of the ball. Bend the legs and pull them forward. Extend the legs back to the start. Torso stays in the same position.	For core stability and balance work. Contract the core muscles to stabilize.	Different arm/leg position. With one or both legs.
Standing Feet on the BOSU. The back is straight. The ball is held by the hands on the upper back. Lean forward at the hips until the body is close to parallel to the floor. Extend the torso back up to an upright position.	A controversial exercise, when performed with a barbbell, but the stability ball is very light. Contract the core muscles to stabilize and keep the back straight throughout the exercise. Neck in neutral. Do not drop the head as this often makes the back round.	With or without resistance. With barbell/dumbbells/a ball.
Standing on the floor in front of the ball. Back leg on the ball, front leg on a stability trainer. Contract the core muscles and keep the torso upright. Bend the front leg into a one-leg squat. Extend the knee. Return to the starting position.	For advanced exercisers. Requires a good balance. Contract the core muscles to stabilize and keep the back straight throughout the exercise.	With or without resistance.
On all fours on the floor. Torso on the ball. Hands on the ball or the floor. Feet on the floor. Rubberband anchored under one leg and under the other foot (of the working leg). Extend the leg backwards. Return with control.	Contract the core muscles to stabilize. Keep the hips level and stable and avoid arching the back. Neck in neutral position.	With or without support of the hands on the floor.

BRIDGE
WITH BARBELL
BRIDGE ON THE BALL

Primary muscles:
Gluteus maximus, hamstrings,
erector spinae, transversus
abdominis, multifidii

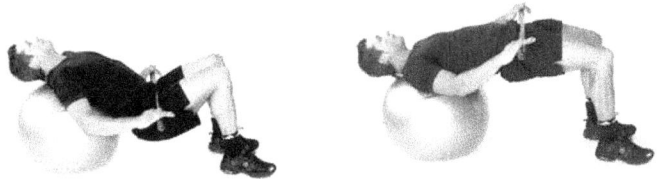

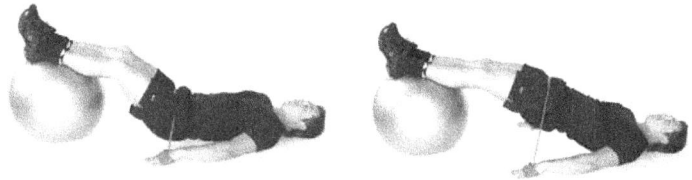

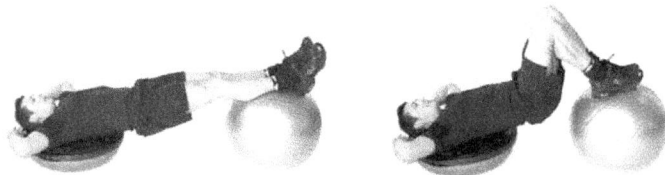

BRIDGE WITH BAND
FEET ON THE BALL
SUPINE ON THE FLOOR

Primary muscles:
Gluteus maximus, hamstrings,
erector spinae, transversus
abdominis, multifidii

HAMSTRING CURL
UNILATERAL
WITH RUBBERBAND/BAND
PRONE ON THE BALL

Primary muscles: Hamstrings,
gluteus maximus, multifidii,
transversus abdominis

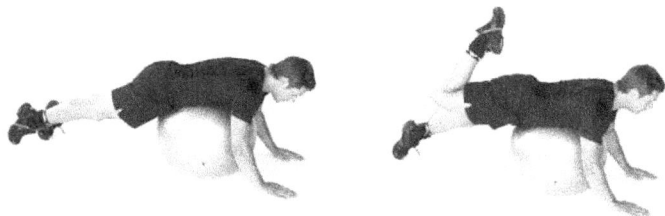

HAMSTRING CURL
WITH THE BALL
SUPINE ON REVERSE BOSU

Primary muscles:
Gluteus maximus, hamstrings,
transversus abdominis,
multifidii

Bridge position on the ball. Feet on the floor hip-wide apart. Upper back on the ball. Bodybar/barbell across the hips. The hands hold the barbell. Contract the buttocks and hamstrings and lift into bridge position. Lower.	Keep the hips level.	Different leg position. With both or one leg.
Supine on the floor. Lower legs on the ball. Band across the hips. Arms on the floor. The hands anchor the ends of the band to the floor. Contract the buttocks and lift into bridge position against the resistance of the band. Lower.	Contract the core muscles to stabilize. Keep the hips level.	With both or one leg on the ball.
Prone on the ball. Feet on the floor. Hands on the ball or on the floor. Rubberband around both ankles or under the foot. Bend the knee of one leg. Return with control. Repeat. After a set change leg.	If possible lift the leg higher into hip extension Contract the core muscles to stabilize. Keep the hips level.	With or without support on the hands.
Supine on a BOSU turned upside down. Arm position optional. Feet on top of the ball. Contract the hamstrings and pull the ball in towards the buttocks. Return to the starting position with control.	Contract the core muscles, avoid arching the lower back. Keep the hips level.	With the BOSU on the other, stable, side (easier). With both or one leg on the ball.

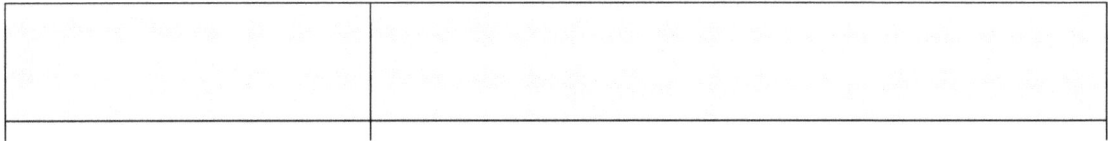

**ABDUCTION
WITH RUBBERBAND/BAND
PRONE ON THE BALL**

Primary muscles:
Gluteus medius and minimus

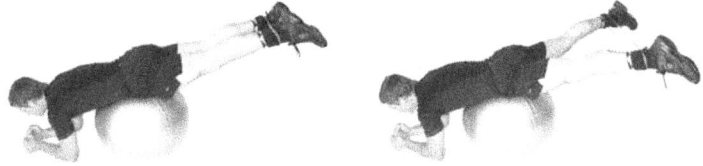

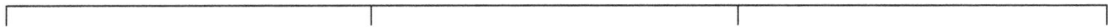

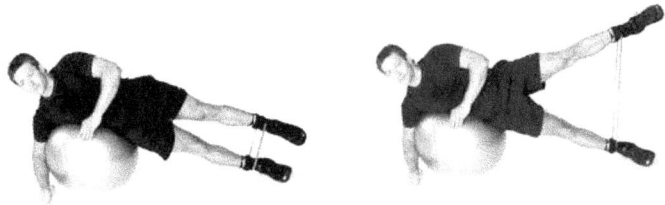

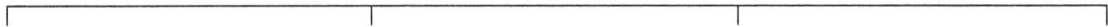

**ABDUCTION
WITH RUBBERBAND/BAND
SIDELYING ON THE BALL**

Primary muscles:
Gluteus medius and minimus

**ADDUCTION
WITH RUBBERBAND/BAND
SIDELYING ON THE BALL**

Primary muscles:
Adductors

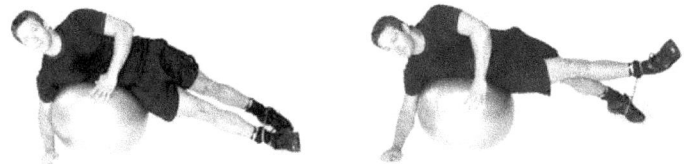

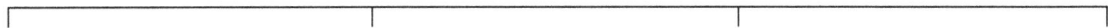

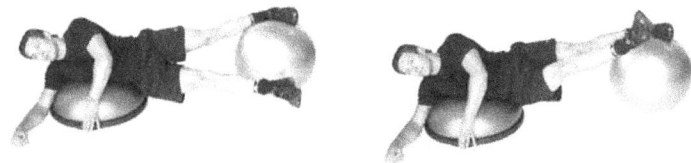

**ADDUCTION
WITH THE BALL
SIDELYING ON A BOSU**

Primary muscles:
Adductors

Prone on the ball. Hands and forearms on the floor. Legs are lifted above horizontal. Rubberband around both ankles. Abduct the legs to the side. Return with control.	Contract the core muscles to stabilize. For balance and abductor work. Keep the tension in the band.	Different body position. The rubberband can be placed above the knee in case of knee problems.
Sidelying on the ball. Bottom hand on the floor or the ball. Top hand on the ball. Hips and legs straight. Bottom foot (side of the foot) on the floor. Top leg lifted just above the bottom leg. Rubberband around both ankles. Abduct the top leg. Lower with control.	Contract the core muscles to stabilize. Keep the tension in the band. The body is on a straight line. Keep the neck neutral, avoid lifting the head up.	Hips and legs straight or slightly bent. With or without hip rotation. The rubberband can be placed above the knee in case of knee problems.
Sidelying on the ball. Top leg slightly bent, foot on the floor behind bottom leg. Bottom leg straight and slightly lifted off the floor. Rubberband anchored under foot on the floor and around working leg ankle. Lift the bottom leg into adduction, past the top leg. Lower.	Contract the core muscles to stabilize. Keep the tension in the band. The body is on a straight line. Keep the neck neutral, avoid lifting the head up.	With one or both legs. With or without hip rotation.
Sidelying on a BOSU. Top leg on top of the ball. Lower leg lifted slightly off the floor and in front of the ball. Lift the lower leg up into adduction. Lower with control.	Contract the core muscles to stabilize.	Working leg knee straight or bent (short or long lever).

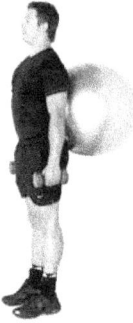

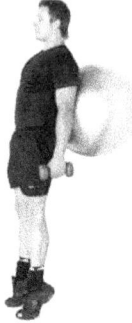

CALF RAISE WITH DUMBBELLS STRAIGHT LEGS, STANDING BY WALL AGAINST BALL Primary muscles: Gastrocnemeus and soleus	
CALF RAISE WITH DUMBBELLS BENT LEGS, STANDING BY WALL AGAINST BALL Primary muscles: Soleus and gastrocnemeus	
CALF RAISE WITH BODYBAR SITTING ON THE BALL Primary muscles: Soleus and gastrocnemeus	
DORSIFLEXION WITH BODYBAR SITTING ON THE BALL Primary muscles: Tibialis anterior	

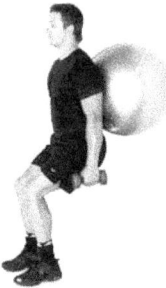

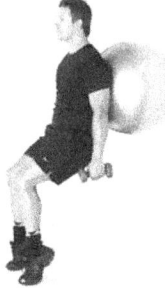

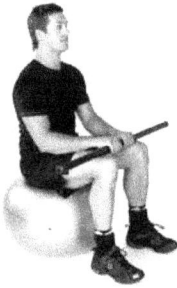

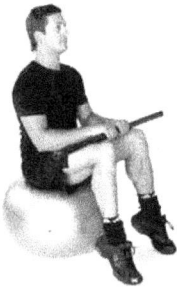

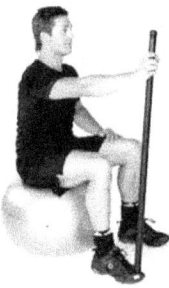

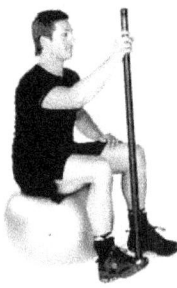

Standing on the floor. Feet on the floor. Legs straight. The back is on the ball, which is pressed against the wall. Arms at sides. Dumbbells in hands. Raise the heels, lift up on the toes. Lower with control.	Contract the core muscles to stabilize.	Different arm position. With one or both legs.
Standing on the floor. Feet on the floor. Legs bent. Back is on the ball, which is pressed against the wall. Arms at sides. Dumbbells in the hands. Raise the heels, lift up on the toes. Lower with control.	Contract the core muscles to stabilize. Keep the knees bent; the body is moved up and down using the calf muscles.	Different arm position. With one or both legs.
Sitting on the ball. Feet on the floor. Barbell across the legs. The hands hold the barbell. Contract the calf muscles and raise the heels. Lower with control.	Contract the core muscles to stabilize.	Different arm position. With one or both legs.
Sitting on the ball. Feet on the floor. One hand holds a barbell, vertical, one end on the toes of one foot. Contract the shin muscles to raise the toes. Lower with control.	Contract the core muscles to stabilize. Be careful: Pressure on top of the foot can pinch the nerves. If it is uncomfortable and a thick sock and shoe does not help, find an alternative exercise.	With or without rubberband/ barbell.

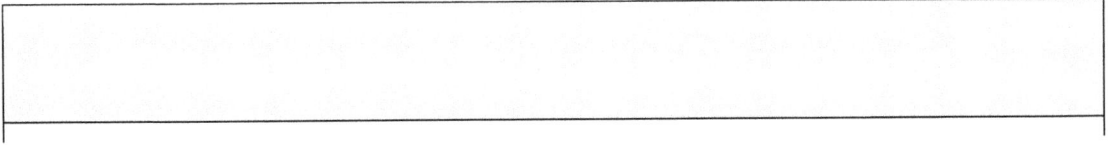

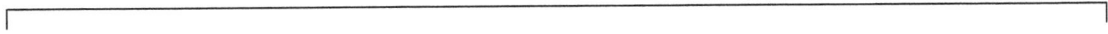

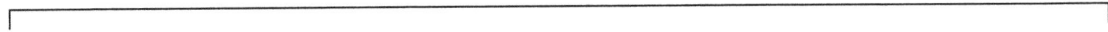

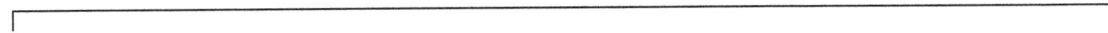

9 | Partner Ball Exercises

Stability ball training with a partner, with or without active use of the stability ball, provides additional exercise options and makes the workout a sociable experience.

In this section you find stability ball exercises for the major muscle groups in the upper and lower body and torso, for two exercisers and one or two balls plus additional equipment.

As partner exercises are new to many exercisers, start with easy exercises and exercises in which you are doing the exercises together but maybe just by sharing the stability ball, so you are not touching each other, but are connected via the ball.

To go on to exercising with a partner, hold or support a partner's, shoulder, elbow, forearm or lower legs, or feet against feet. Eventually add exercises holding hands or leaning on or lifting one another.

Focus points:

- Same height and weight – approximately.
- Equal strength – approximately.
- Clear communication between each other.
- Agree upon when to start, so that both are ready.
- Synchronized movements – both work at the same speed.
- A partner initially only support or oppose – later on apply force with control and care.
- Hold or support over or under a joint, never directly on the joint.
- Limit periods, where one partner is inactive. Keep the intensity, so exercise sets, where one partner just assists seem timely and appropriate. Take turns to perform sets, so that no exerciser feels that he or she is wasting time.

Important: All exercises are for healthy exercisers free from any serious or disabilitating disease, illness or ailments. Please consult your doctor before beginning these exercises.

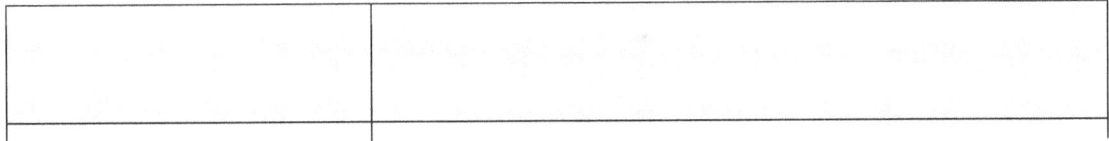

**CHEST PUSH-UP
PLANK POSITION
HANDS ON THE BALL**

Primary muscles:
Pectoralis major, anterior
deltoid, triceps brachii,
transversus abd., multifidii

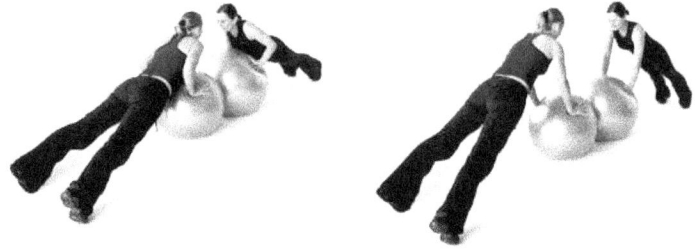

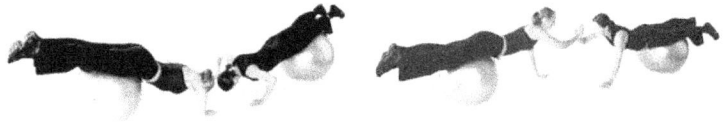

**PUSH-UP WITH CLAP
PLANK POSITION
LEGS ON THE BALL**

Primary muscles:
Pectoralis major, anterior
deltoid, triceps brachii,
transversus abd., multifidii

**PUSH-UP ON THE BALL
LEG PRESS WITH THE BALL
STANDING/SUPINE**

Primary muscles:
Torso- and leg-muscles,
transversus abominis, multidii

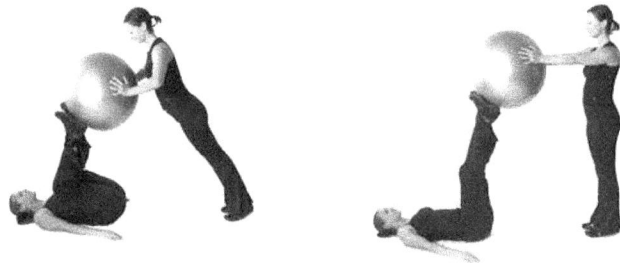

**PULLOVER ON THE BALL
WITH RESISTANCE BAND
SUPINE ON THE BALL**

Primary muscles:
Pectoralis major, deltoids,
latissimus dorsi, transversus
abdominis, multifidii

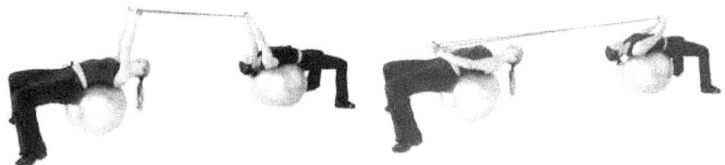

Plank position. Toes on the floor. Hands on the ball. Balls against each other. Bend the arms and lower the body down towards the ball. Extend the arms to push the body back up again.	Neck, shoulder girdle and lower back in neutral position. As a traditionel push-up on the ball, but in this exercise you can lean more into the stability ball.	Different arm/leg position. Feet wide apart (easier) or together (difficult). May be performed kneeling behind the ball (easiest version).
Plank position. Hands on the floor. Thighs on the ball. Partners face each other. Bend the arms, lower the body towards the floor. Extend the arms, push up again and clap the hand of the partner. Repeat with the opposite hand.	Neck, shoulder girdle and lower back in neutral position.	Different arm/leg position. On the hip, thighs, lower legs or the feet depending on the desired level of difficulty.
Standing and supine. The ball is held between the hands of one partner and the feet of the other partner. The supine partner extends the legs, while the standing partner bends and extends the arms (push-up). After a set the partners change place.	Start carefully; coordinate resistance and tempo. Make sure the ball is kept in place between the hands and the feet, so the standing exerciser does not fall. Minimal strengthening effect, but nice balance, coordination and core exercise.	Different arm/body position.
Supine on the ball. Feet on the floor. Facing away from each other. Arms straight and back overhead. Ends of the band in the hands. Bands looped around each other. Contract the back and chest muscles and pull the arms over the head and forward over the torso. Return with control.	As you are supine and face away from each other, there is no visual contact. Therefore initially count out loud, so you pull at the same time. In partner band exercises it is important, that you pull at the same time.	Different body/leg position. With tube or band.

**CHEST FLY, UNILATERAL
WITH RESISTANCE BAND
SITTING ON THE BALL**

Primary muscles:
Pectoralis major, deltoids
anterior, transversus
abdominis, multifidii

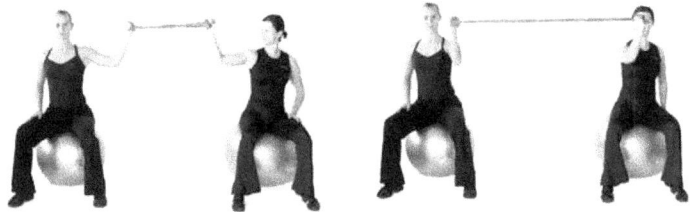

**CHEST PRESS
WITH RESISTANCE BAND
SITTING ON THE BALL**

Primary muscles:
Pectoralis major, triceps
brachii, anterior deltoid,
transversus abd., multifidii

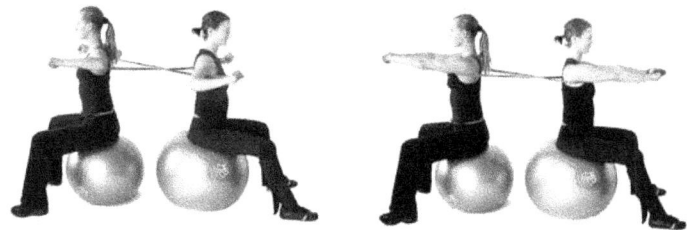

**SHOULDER, UNILATERAL
LATERAL ROTATION
WITH RESISTANCE BAND
SITTING ON THE BALL**

Primary muscles:
Infraspinatus, transversus
abdominis, multifidii

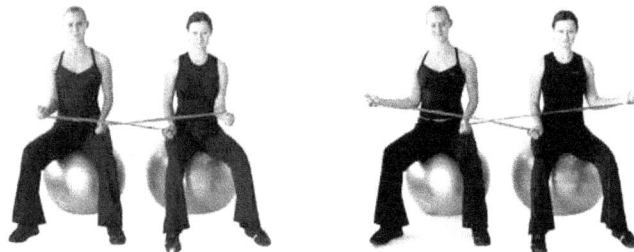

**SHOULDER, UNILATERAL
MEDIAL ROTATION
WITH RESISTANCE BAND
SITTING ON THE BALL**

Primary muscles:
Subscapularis, transversus
abdominis, multifidii

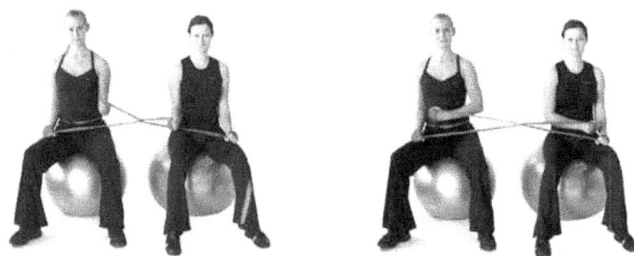

Sitting on the ball. Feet on the floor. Sitting side by side. The band in the inside hand. Bands looped around each other. Upper arm to the side in horizontal, elbow bent. Contract the chest muscles to adduct the arm in front of the torso. Return with control. Change side.	Because the anchorpoint of the rubberband moves, the line of action is not optimal in this exercise. Keep the torso stable. Movement is in the shoulder. In partner resistance band exercises it is important, that you press at the same time.	Different arm/body position. With or without support, feet on the floor or lifted off the floor.
Sitting on the ball. Feet on the floor. Facing away from each other. Ends of the band in the hands. Bands looped around each other behind the body. Arms to the side, elbows bent. Press the arms straight forward, until the arms are straight with hands together. Return with control.	Keep the torso stable. As you are sitting back to back, there is no visual contact. Therefore initially count out loud, so you press at the same time.	Different arm/body position. **CHEST FLY** Arms slightly bent and to the side in horizontal plane. Adduct the ams in front of the torso with no movement in the elbows. Return with control. Note: The line of action is not optimal.
Sitting on the ball. Feet on the floor. Sitting side by side. The band is in the outside hand. Bands are looped around each other and anchored by the inside hand. The arm is bent 90 degrees, elbow by the side. Rotate the outside arm out away from the midline of the body. Return with control.	Contract the core muscles. In partner resistance band exercises it is important, that you pull at the same time. After a set change side or perform medial rotation with the opposite arm. Then change side.	Different leg position. With tube or band.
Sitting on the ball. Feet on the floor. Sitting side by side. Band in the inside hand. Bands are looped around each other and anchored by the outside hand. The arm is bent 90 degrees, elbow by the side. Rotate the inside arm in front of the torso. Return. Change side.	Contract the core muscles. In partner resistance band exercises it is important, that you pull at the same time to make the exercise work. After a set perform lateral rotation with the opposite arm. Then change side (ball).	Different leg position. With tube or band.

ROWING, NARROW,
WITH RESISTANCE BAND
SITTING ON THE BALL

Primary muscles:
Latissimus dorsi, posterior
deltoid, biceps brachii,
transversus abd., multifidii

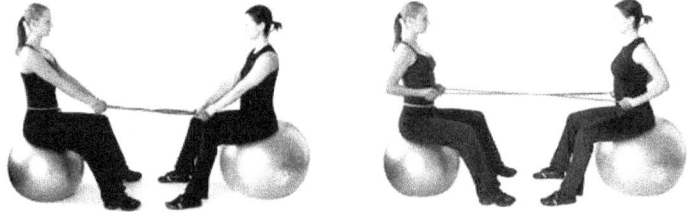

ROWING, WIDE,
WITH RESISTANCE BAND
SITTING ON THE BALL

Primary muscles:
Rhomboids, posterior deltoid,
biceps brachii, transversus
abdominis, multifidii

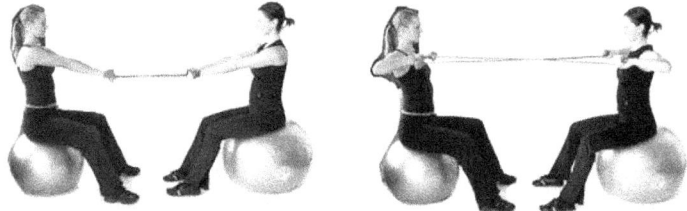

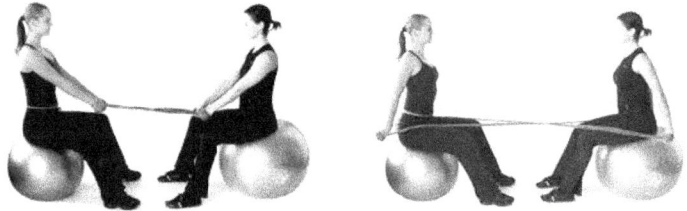

LAT PULL, STRAIGHT ARMS,
WITH RESISTANCE BAND
SITTING ON THE BALL

Primary muscles:
Rhomboids, posterior deltoid,
transversus abdominis,
multifidii

LAT PULL
WITH RESISTANCE BAND
PRONE ON THE BALL

Primary muscles:
Latissimus dorsi, deltoids,
biceps brachii, erector spinae,
transversus abd., multifidii

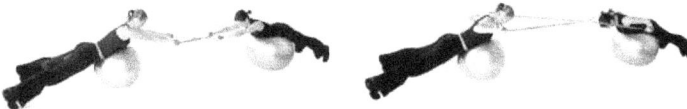

Sitting on the ball. Feet on the floor. Facing each other. Ends of the band in the hands. Bands are looped around each other. Arms forward. Pull the arms back, closely past the torso, sagittal plane, until the elbows are bent and behind the body, hands at the waist. Return with control.	In partner resistance band exercises it is important, that you pull at the same time to make the exercise work. Keep the torso erect.	Different arm/body position. With or without support, the feet on the floor or lifted off the floor. With tube or band.
Sitting on the ball. The feet on the floor. Front to each other. Ends of the band in the hands. Bands are looped around each other. Arms forward. Pull the arms back in horizontal plane, at chest level. The elbows lead. Adduct the shoulder blades in the end position. Return with control.	In partner resistance band exercises it is important, that you pull at the same time to make the exercise work. Keep the torso erect.	Different arm/body position. With or without support, the feet on the floor or lifted off the floor. With tube or band.
Sitting on the ball. Facing each other. Ends of the band in the hands. Bands are looped around each other. Arms straight and forward. Pull the arms back closely past the body, until the straight arms are behind the body. Return with control.	In partner resistance band exercises it is important, that you pull at the same time to make the exercise work. Keep the torso erect.	Different leg position. With tube or band.
Prone on the ball. Toes on the floor. Face each other. Ends of the band in the hands. Bands are looped around each other. Arms forward. Pull the arms back and down, bend the arms and bring the upper arms close to torso and hands by the shoulders. Return with contol.	Neck in neutral position, look down or diagonally forward. Do not drop the head or look up. In partner resistance band exercises it is important, that you pull at the same time to make the exercise work.	Different leg position. With tube or band.

**BICEPS CURL WITH
RESISTANCE BAND
SUPINE ON THE BALL**

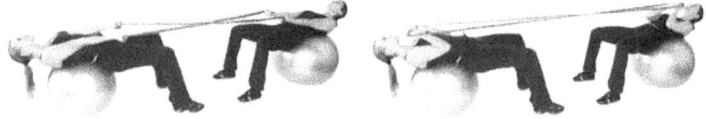

Primary muscles:
Biceps brachii, transversus
abdominis, multifidii,
gluteus maximus, hamstrings

**TRICEPS KICK BACK
WITH RESISTANCE BAND
PRONE ON THE BALL**

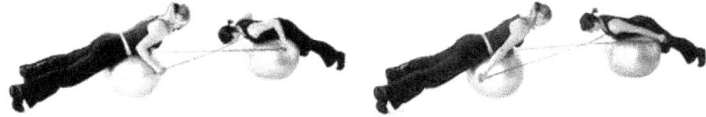

Primary muscles:
Triceps brachii, transversus
abdominis, multifidii,
erector spinae

**'UPRIGHT' ROWING
WITH BAND
SUPINE ON THE BALL**

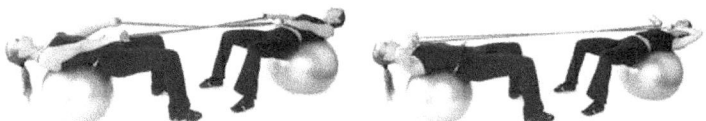

Primary muscles:
Deltoids, transversus
abdominis, multifidii

**LATERAL RAISE
WITH RESISTANCE BAND
SUPINE ON THE BALL**

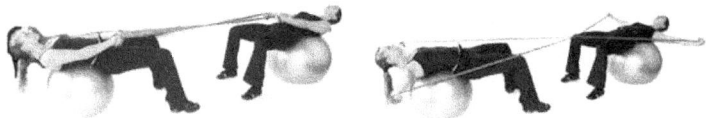

Primary muscles:
Deltoids, transversus
abdominis, multifidii

Supine on the ball. Feet on the floor. Face each other. Ends of the band in the hands. Bands are looped around each other. Arms at sides. Underhand grip. Bend the arms, forearm curl up, until the hands are close to the shoulders. Return with control.	In partner resistance band exercises it is important, that you pull at the same time to make the exercise work. The elbows flex and extend completely, without hyper-extending, for full range of motion. Avoid too small a range of motion in this exercise.	Different arm/body/leg position. Lie in bridge position for added resistance training or on the back for support. With tube or band.
Prone on the ball. Feet on the floor. Face each other. Ends of the band in the hands. Bands are looped around each other. Upper arms close to the torso. Extend the elbows, straighten the arms. Elbows remain in the same position throughout the exercise. Return with control.	In partner resistance band exercises it is important, that you pull at the same time to make the exercise work. Extend the elbows completely, without hyper-extending, to have full range of motion. Avoid too small a range of motion in this exercise.	Different arm/body/leg position. With tube or band.
Supine on the ball. Feet on the floor. Face each other. Bands are looped around each other. Ends of the band in the hands. Arms straight and down in front of the body. Overhand grip. Pull the arms upwards in front of the torso, elbows lead, hands close to the collarbone. Return with control.	Contract the core muscles. In partner resistance band exercises it is important, that you pull at the same time to make the exercise work.	Different arm/body/leg position. With tube or band. Lie in bridge position for added resistance training. Hold the hands together or apart throughout the exercise.
Supine on the ball. Feet on the floor. Face each other. Ends of the band in the hands. Bands are looped around each other. Arms are straight and at sides. Neutral grip. Raise, abduct, the arms straight to the side, frontal plane, until the arms are at shoulder level. Return with control.	Contract the core to stabilize. In partner resistance band exercises it is important, that you pull at the same time to make the exercise work. The arms are almost straight, elbows relaxed.	Different arm/body/leg position. Lie in bridge position for added resistance training. With tube or band.

AB CURL
SUPINE ON THE FLOOR
LEGS ON ONE BALL

Primary muscles:
Rectus abdominis,
obliques externus and internus

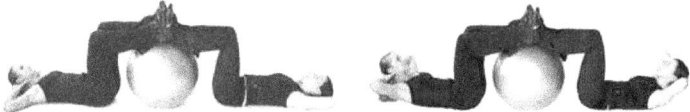

AB CURL
SUPINE ON THE FLOOR
LEGS HOLDING ONE BALL

Primary muscles:
Rectus abdominis,
obliques externus and
internus, quadriceps

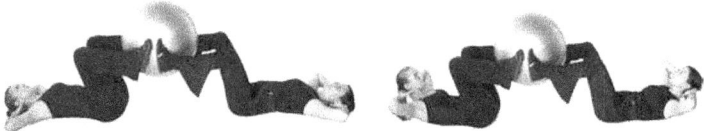

SIT UP/REVERSE CURL
WITH BALL PASS
SUPINE ON THE FLOOR

Primary muscles:
Rectus abdominis, obliques
externus and internus,
transversus abdominis

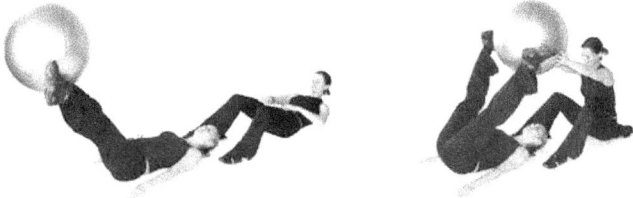

BALL PASS
OVER AND UNDER
STANDING ON THE FLOOR

Primary muscles:
Erector spinae, rectus
abdominis, obliques

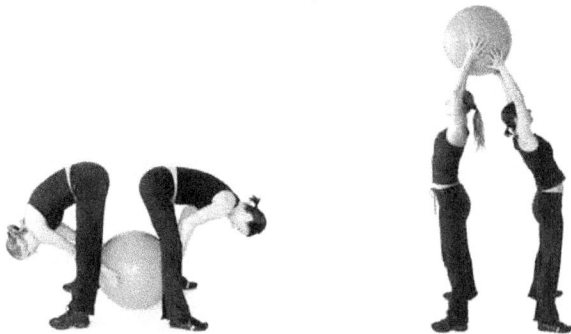

Supine on the floor. One ball between the partners. Lower legs of both partners on top of the ball. Contract the abdominals and curl the torso up. Lower with control.	Not a true partner exercise, where you depend on each other, but sharing the stability ball provides a social element. The feet may or may not touch. An option in group exercise classes with not enough balls for all participants.	Different arm/body position.
Supine on the floor. One ball between the feet of both partners. Feet on the side of the ball holding it up, off the floor. Contract the abdominals and curl torso up. Lower.	Not a true partner exercise, where you depend on each other, but sharing the stability ball provides a social element. The feet may or may not touch. An option in group exercise classes with not enough balls for all participants.	Different arm/body position.
Supine on the floor. Face the same way. Back partner does a sit up with ball in hands. Front partner does a reverse ab curl with straight legs and takes the ball with the feet in top position. Both lower down, curl back up, and back partner takes the ball again. Both lower. Repeat.	Not a true partner exercise, where you depend on each other, but sharing the stability ball provides a social element. The stability ball works as a light dumbbell, approx. 1-1.5 kg, in this exercise.	Different arm/leg position.
Standing on the floor. Feet wide apart. Face away from each other and stand a little apart. One has the ball in the hands. Both bend down. The ball is passed through the legs to the other partner. Both return to upright position. Back extension, pass the ball overhead. Repeat.	A fun coordination exercise with extension and flexion of the spine. Mobility work for the spine. Start with a slow tempo.	Different leg position. Perform with a medicine ball for added resistance.

**OBLIQUE CURL
SUPINE ON THE FLOOR
LEGS ON ONE BALL**

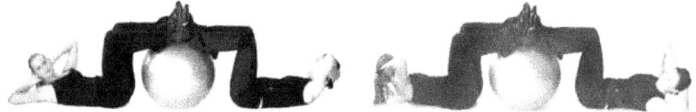

Primary muscles:
Rectus abdominis,
obliques externus and internus

**OBLIQUE CURL
SUPINE ON THE FLOOR
LEGS HOLD ONE BALL**

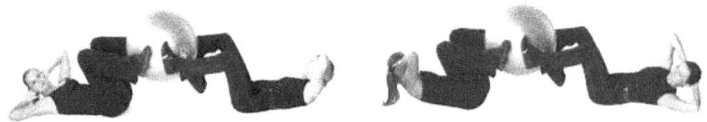

Primary muscles:
Obliques externus and
internus, transversus
abdominis, multifidii

**TORSO ROTATION
AND BALL PASS
SITTING ON THE FLOOR**

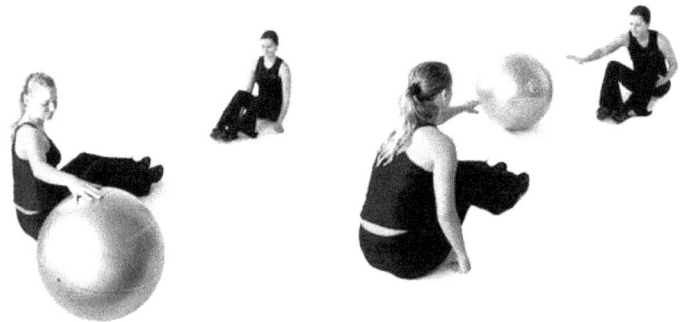

Primary muscles:
Obliques externus and
internus, transversus
abdominis, multifidii

**TORSO ROTATION
AND BALL PASS
SITTING ON THE BALL**

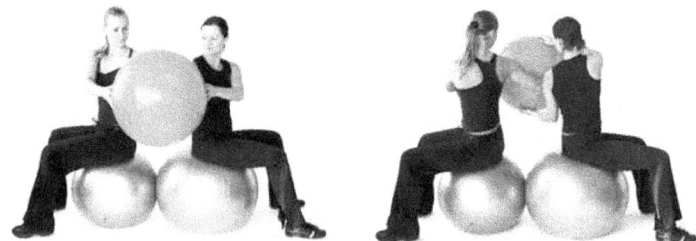

Primary muscles:
Obliques externus and
internus, transversus
abdominis, multifidii

Supine on the floor. One ball between the partners. Lower legs of both partners on top of the ball. Feet together. Hands at the chest or by the side of the head. Contract the abdominals and curl up and twist to the right. Lower and repeat to the left.	Not a true partner exercise, where you depend on each other, but sharing the stability ball provides a social element. An option in group exercise with not enough balls for all participants.	Different arm/body position. Perform a set to one side and then a set to the other side. Or alternate from side to side.
Supine on the floor. One ball between the feet of both partners. The lower legs are on the sides of the ball holding it up off the floor. Hands by the side of the head. Contract the abdominals and curl up and twist to the right. Lower and repeat to the left.	Not a true partner exercise, where you depend on each other, but sharing the stability ball provides a social element. An option in group exercise with not enough balls for all participants.	Different arm/body position. Hands at the chest or by the side of the head. Perform a set to one side and then a set to the other side. Or alternate from side to side.
Sitting on the floor. Some distance apart. Face each other. Roll the ball to the partner, who rolls the ball behind and around the body. Roll the balll back to the partner, who rolls the ball behind and around the body. Repeat. Repeat the opposite way.	Easy coordination and core work. Contract the core muscles.	Different leg position.
Sitting on a ball. Two balls close together. The partners sit back to back, facing away from each other. Both turn to the same side to pass and receive the ball respectively. Repeat 4-8 times. Repeat 4-8 times the opposite way around.	Easy coordination and core work. Contract the core muscles. In time perform the exercise unsupported, with the feet lifted off the floor.	Different leg position.

**TORSO ROTATION
AND BALL PASS
STANDING ON THE FLOOR**

Primary muscles:
Obliques externus and
internus, transversus
abdominis, multifidii

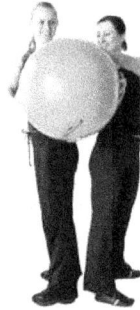

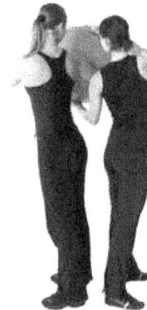

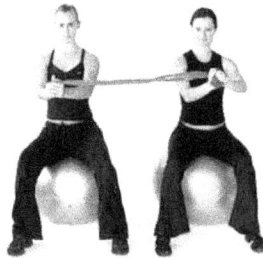

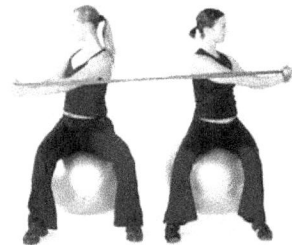

**TORSOROTATION
WITH RESISTANCE BAND
SITTING ON THE BALL**

Primary muscles:
Obliques externus and
internus, transversus
abdominis, multifidii

**SIDEBEND
FEET ANCHORED
SIDELYING ON THE BALL**

Primary muscles:
Quadratus lomborum,
obliques, transversus
abdominis, multifidii

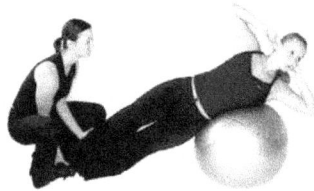

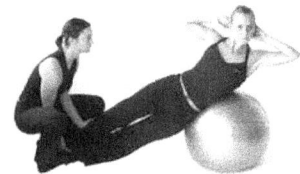

**TURNING BODIES
WITH BALL
STANDING ON THE FLOOR**

Primary muscles:
Transversus abdominis,
multifidii, erector spinae

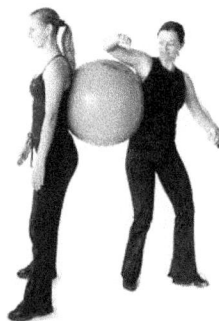

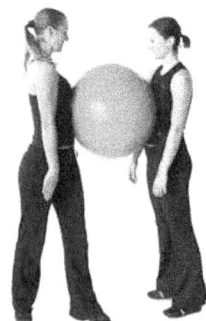

Standing on the floor. Back to back. Face away from each other. Partners turn towards each other to pass and receive the stability ball respectively. Repeat 4-8 times. Repeat 4-8 times the opposite way.	Easy coordination and core work. Contract the core muscles.	Different leg position. Perform with a medicine ball for added resistance.
Sitting on the ball. Side by side. Bands are looped around each other. Arms are bent and in front of the body. Hands together and band in hands. Arms and hands remain in the same position throughout the exercise. Contract the obliques and rotate away from partner. Return with control. Repeat.	Keep the torso upright and rotate to the side. Focus on deep slow breathing. In partner resistance band exercises it is important, that you pull at the same time to make the exercise work. After a set change side and repeat the exercise.	Different arm/leg position. With tube or band.
Sidelying on the ball. One partner holds the lower legs/legs anchored. Arms are at the chest or by the side of the head. Contract and lift the torso sideways (deep ab muscles). Lower. Repeat opposite side.	Partners change place after each side – or each set, so one partner is not having too long a rest.	Different arm/leg position.
Standing on the floor. Side by side. The ball is held in place between the partners by pressing into the ball. Both partners turn around themselves, while trying to keep the ball in place, so it does not fall. Repeat turning the opposite way.	Coordination exercise.	Different leg position. Start by facing each other or stand side by side facing away from each other.

V-SIT, LEG PRESS (SAW)
SITTING ON THE FLOOR

Primary muscles:
Rectus abdominis, obliques,
iliopsoas, quadriceps,
transversus abdominis,
multifidii

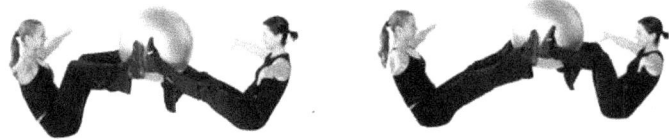

RAINBOW
SUPINE ON THE FLOOR

Primary muscles:
Obliques externus and
internus, erector spinae,
transverses abdominis,
multifidii

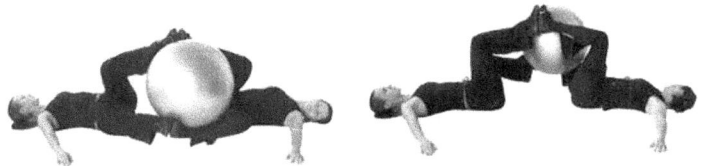

AB CURL
WITH RESISTANCE BAND
SUPINE ON THE BALL

Primary muscles:
Rectus abdominis,
obliques, transversus
abdominis, multifidii

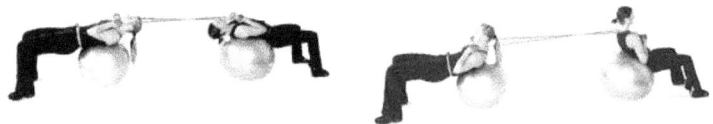

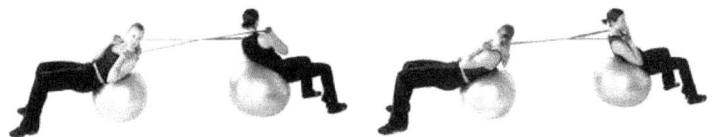

OBLIQUE CURL
WITH RESISTANCE BAND
SUPINE ON THE BALL

Primary muscles:
Rectus abdominis,
obliques, transversus
abdominis, multifidii

Sitting in balance on the floor, V-sit, facing each other. Arms down or to the side to keep the balance. Legs are lifted off the floor. The ball is held between the feet of both partners. One partner stretches the legs, while the other partner bends the legs. Alternate.	Keep the core muscles contracted to hold the body stable. Sharing the stability ball provides a social element and an element of coordination.	Different arm/body position.
Supine on the floor. Hips and legs bent 90 degrees. The ball is lifted off the floor and held between the feet of both partners. Arms on the floor to stabilize. Contract the obliques and lower the ball one side. Return to neutral. Repeat to the opposite side.	Oblique exercise; start with a small range of motion to protect the spine. Increase range of motion very gradually. Contract the core muscles to stabilize. Coordinate the movement tempo.	Different leg position. Legs are bent (or straight). Perform with a medicine ball for increased resistance.
Supine on the ball. Both partners on a ball, back to back, some distance apart. Arms bent, hands by the shoulders. Bands are looped around each other. The ends of the band in the hands. Contract the abs and curl up. Lower with control.	Contract the core muscles to stabilize. Neck in neutral position. In partner resistance band exercises it is important, that you pull at the same time to make the exercise work. Count out loud to coordinate.	Different arm/body position. With tube or band.
Supine on the ball. Both partners on a ball, back to back, some distance apart. Hands by the shoulders. Bands are looped around each other. The ends of the band in the hands. Contract the obliques and curl up and twist to the right at the same time. Lower. Repeat left.	Contract the core muscles to stabilize. Neck in neutral position. In partner resistance band exercises it is important, that you pull at the same time to make the exercise work. Count out loud to coordinate.	Different arm/body position. With tube or band.

SQUAT
BACK TO BACK
BALL BETWEEN PARTNERS
STANDING ON THE FLOOR

Primary muscles:
Gluteus maximus, hamstrings,
quadriceps

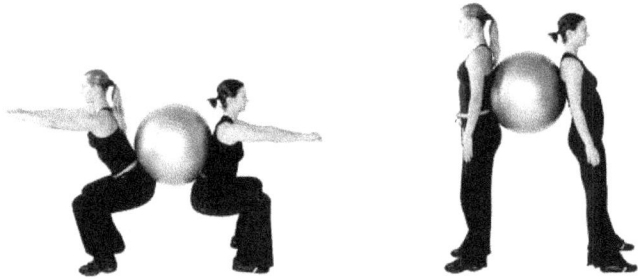

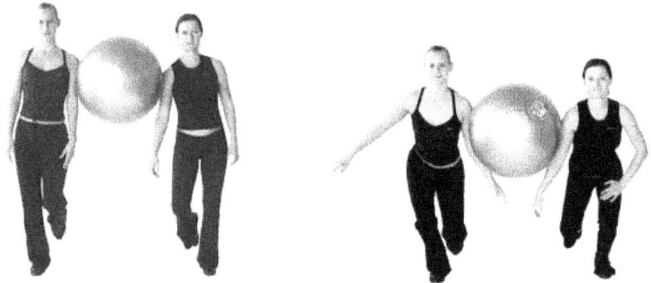

ONE-LEG SQUAT
SIDE BY SIDE
BALL BETWEEN PARTNERS
STANDING ON THE FLOOR

Primary muscles:
Gluteus maximus, hamstrings,
quadriceps

BODY PRESS
STANDING ON THE FLOOR

Primary muscles:
Total body exercise – focus on
isometric strength, balance
and coordination

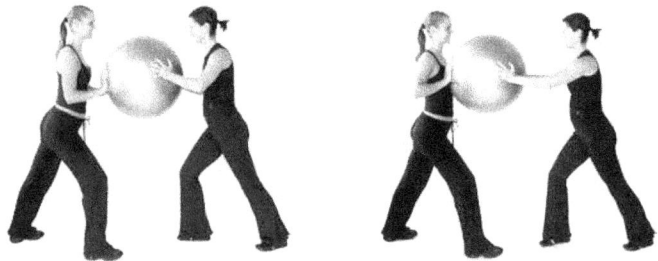

BALANCE
BALL PLAY
SITTING ON THE BALL

Primary muscles:
Transversus abdominis,
multifidii, the legmuscles

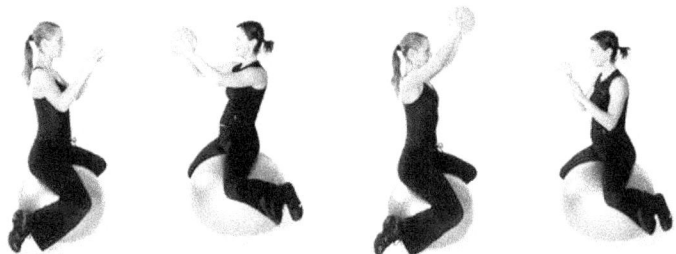

Standing on the floor. Back to back. The ball is between the backs. Lean against the stability ball. Bend the legs into a squat. Extend the legs back up; keep contracting the leg muscles, do not relax in the top position.	The exercisers should be of approximately the same height and weight. Slow tempo, until you get the hang of the exercise. As there is no visual contact, talk to each other and coordinate the movement.	Different leg position.
Standing on the floor. Stand on the outside leg, inside leg is lifted. Side by side. The ball is anchored between the upper arms of the partners. Lean carefully into the stability ball. Bend outside leg down into a one-leg squat. Extend the leg. After a set repeat with the opposite leg.	The exercisers should be of approximately the same height and weight. Slow tempo, until you get the hang of the exercise. Lean carefully into the ball – not too much pressure, if the ball should slip away.	Different leg position.
Standing on the floor facing each other. Staggered feet. Both have the right foot in front. The ball is between the partners, hands on the ball. Both push at the same time trying to push the ball and partner away. After a while, ½-2 minutes, repeat with left leg in front.	The exercisers should be of approximately the same height and weight. Slow tempo, until you get the hang of the exercise. Contract the core muscles to stabilize.	Different arm/body/leg position.
Sitting on the ball. Both partners on a ball facing each other. The feet are lifted off the floor. Keep the balance. Throw a ball to the partner, catch it on return.	For intermediate to advanced exercisers. For balance and coordination. Contract the core muscles to stabilize.	Different arm/body/leg position. Both partners can sit on a ball or one can stand on the floor and throw the ball or push at the partner to challenge the balance.

BALANCE
SITTING ON THE BALL

Primary muscles:
Transversus abdominis,
multifidii, leg muscles

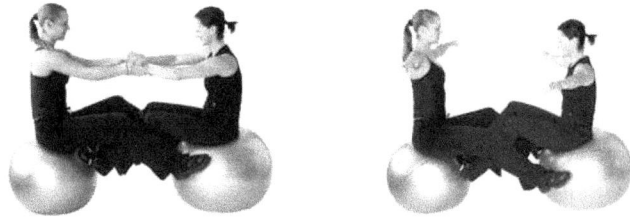

MULTI-BALANCE
WITH BALL, 'MIRROR'
STANDING ON THE FLOOR

Primary muscles:
Total body exercise – focus on
balance and coordination

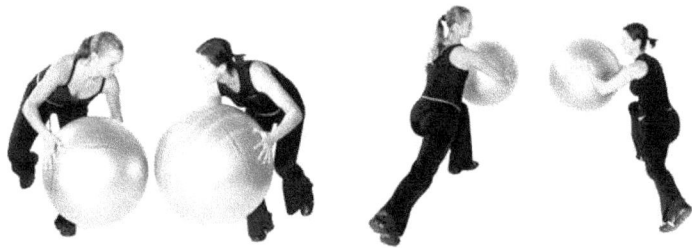

PASS THE BALL
SITTING ON THE FLOOR

Primary muscles:
Upper body muscles and
eye-hand coordination

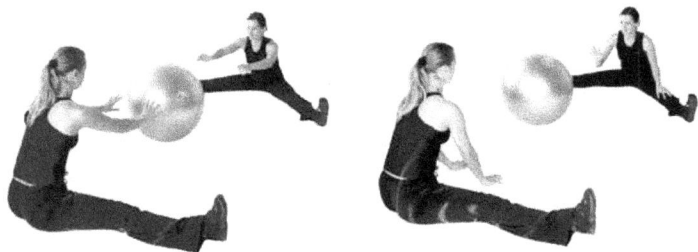

PLAY BALL
STANDING ON THE FLOOR

Primary muscles:
Total body exercise – focus on
balance and eye-hand
coordination

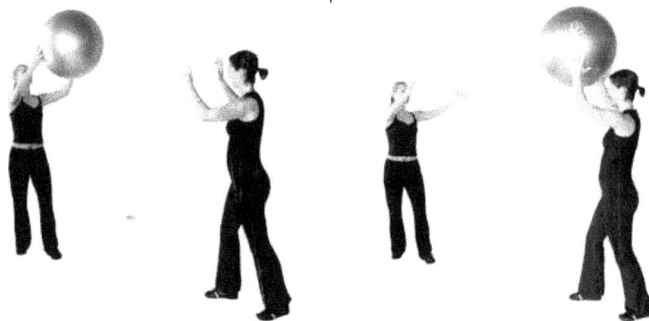

Sitting on the ball. Both partners on a ball facing each other. Legs bent. Both partners have their feet on the ball of the partner. One partner with the legs together, the other with the legs apart, feet wide apart on the ball. Change leg position.	For beginning to advanced exercisers. Balance exercise. Contract the core muscles to stabilize.	Different arm/body/leg position. Hold hands or keep the arms out to the side.
Standing on the floor facing each other. Both have a ball in the hands. One partner moves the body and the ball in various patterns to challenge the balance and coordination. The partner mirrors the moves. Change after a while; the other partner leads.	Coordination and balance. Contract the core muscles to stabilize. Controlled, slow movements, so you are able to follow the lead.	Different arm/body/leg position.
Sitting on the floor. Facing each other, some distance apart. Roll or throw the stability ball to the partner and catch it on return.	Use the stability ball with care: Do not throw or kick it hard or uncontrolled, as if it hits any sharp edges, it may puncture.	Different arm/body/leg position. Standing or kneeling. With balls in different sizes. Walk, run or hop (as in sports games). Add dribbling the ball, before passing the ball back.
Standing on the floor facing each other. Throw the stability ball to the partner and catch it on return. Add walk, jog or jumps.	Use the stability ball with care: Do not throw or kick it hard or uncontrolled; if it hits any sharp edges, it may puncture	Different arm/body/leg position. With balls in different sizes, or a medicine ball. Add dribbling the ball, before passing the ball back.

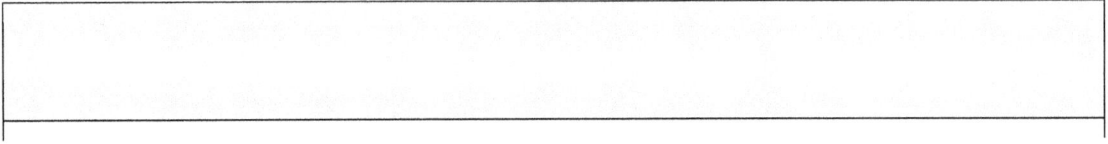

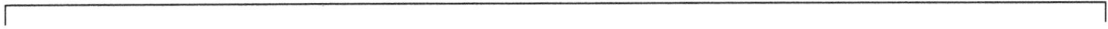

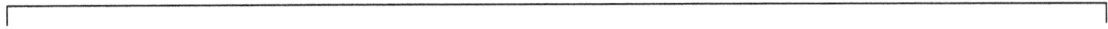

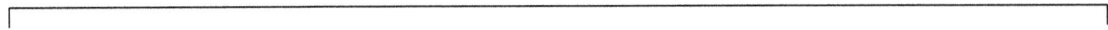

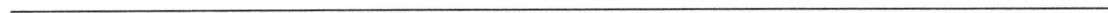

10 | Stability Ball Stretches

Stretching with the stability ball is an excellent supplement or alternative to stretching without the ball. The advantage of the stability ball is that it is soft and comfortable, gives way to the body and facilitates a larger range of motion in many stretches.
It also allows you to perform some stretches, which cannot be performed without the ball.

For an optimal stretching experience, you should relax physically and mentally. The body should be stable and centered, so the muscles do not contract to keep the balance.
In some stretches with the stability ball, you can have a double effect: Stretching one muscle group, while working the balance and stability of other muscles.

For stretching use a ball that is not fully inflated; then it is more stable and do not roll around too much.
However, a slight rolling of the ball is an advantage: Roll the body slightly to stretch the torso and body parts from different angles, *multi-angular stretching*.

At the next pages you find stretches on and with the stability ball. They are essentially organized from 'top to toe', not according to stretching workout sequence. The primary muscles being stretched are listed, and in some exercises also the the stabilizing muscles.

The stretches should be performed slowly and with flow, so you enter each stretch without losing balance and have time to feel how the muscles are being stretched.
When you are in the desired position, make sure that the body and ball is stable. Then relax the mind and body.

The stretches can be short, 15-18 seconds, for an easy stretch, or longer, 30-60 seconds or more, for increased flexibility and relaxation. Short stretches may be repeated 1-4 times.

During the stretches breathe deeply and slowly through the nose; this will relax you even more. Let the stretches follow the breathing; feel the flow of air and movement.

**TRICEPS STRETCH
SITTING ON THE BALL**

Primary muscles:
Triceps brachii

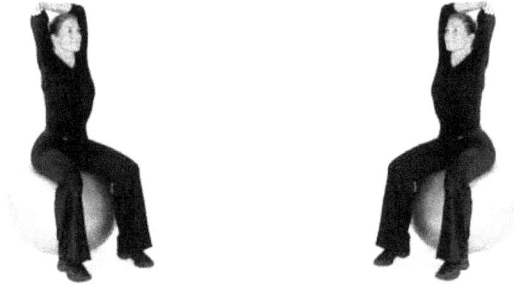

**BICEPS STRETCH
(MORE VARIATIONS)
SITTING ON THE BALL**

Primary muscles:
Biceps brachii,
pectoralis major,
anterior deltoid

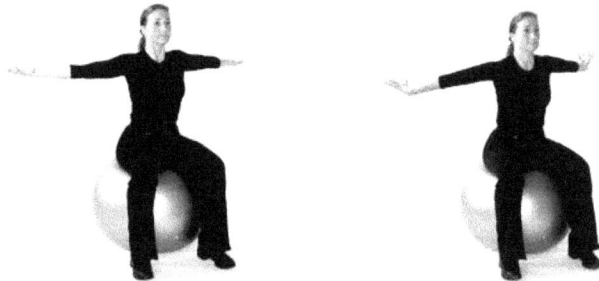

**FOREARM STRETCH
PRONE ON THE BALL**

Primary muscles:
Wrist flexors

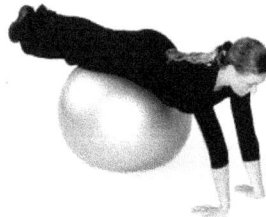

**FINGERSTRETCH
SITTING ON THE BALL
(MORE VARIATIONS)**

Primary muscles:
Finger flexors and
finger extensors

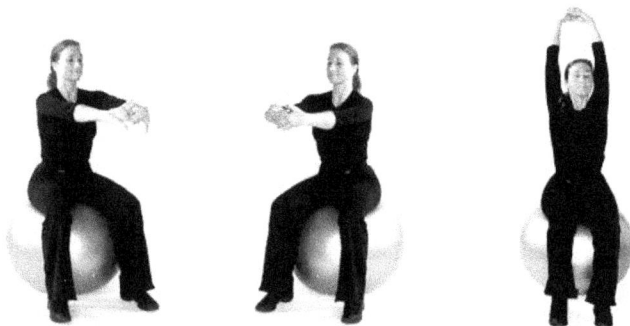

Sitting on the ball. Feet on floor hip-width apart. One arm vertical, elbow bent and forearm behind the head, the hand reaching towards the same side shoulder blade. Opposite hand on the stretch arm to add a slight pressure to increase the triceps stretch. Repeat with the opposite arm.	Focus on deep slow breathing. Stretching on the ball will add an element of balance work.	Different arm/body/leg position. Move the arm in different angles for different stretches. Lean to the side for an increased latissimus dorsi stretch.
Sitting on the ball. Feet on the floor hip-width apart. Both arms out to the side, as far behind the body as possible. Thumbs point down or back to stretch the biceps.	Focus on deep slow breathing. Stretching on the ball will add an element of balance work.	Different arm/body/leg position. Move the arms at different angles and turn the hands up and down for different stretches.
Prone on the ball. Palms on the floor. Fingertips towards the body and the ball. Note: Only a light pressure on the hands and wrists. Thighs on the ball, legs together and lifted off the floor. Carefully roll a little backwards on the ball to stretch the forearms.	Avoid supporting all of the bodyweight on the hands. Move the body back on the ball. Contract the core muscles to stabilize. Neck in neutral position. Focus on deep slow breathing.	Different arm/body/leg position.
Sitting on the stability ball. Feet on the floor. Arms forward. Fingers interlaced, palms turned towards the body, pull the hands away from the body. Then turn the palms away from the body, press the hands forward.	Move the arms in different angles and turn the palms out and in for different stretches. Focus on deep slow breathing. Stretching on the ball will add an element of balance work.	Different arm/body/leg position. Arms behind or in front of the body or overhead.

POSTERIOR DELTOID STRETCH
ARM ON THE BALL
KNEELING ON THE FLOOR

Primary muscles:
Posterior deltoid,
latissimus dorsi

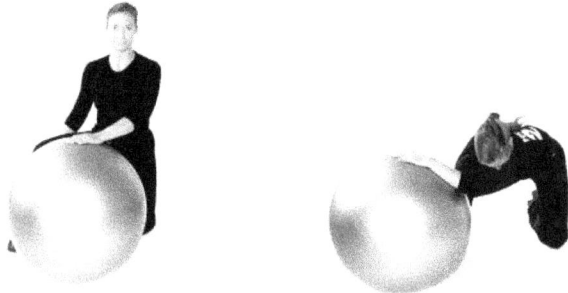

ANTERIOR DELTOID STRETCH
PALM ON THE BALL
KNEELING ON THE FLOOR

Primary muscles:
Anterior deltoid,
pectoralis major,
biceps brachii

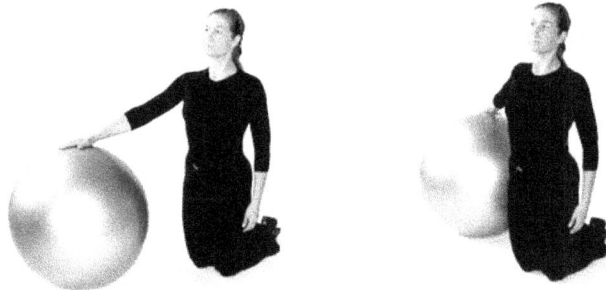

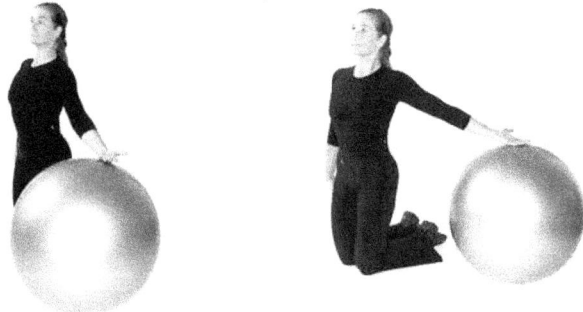

ANTERIOR DELTOID STRETCH
BACK OF HAND ON THE BALL
KNEELING ON THE FLOOR

Primary muscles:
Anterior deltoid, pectoralis
major, biceps brachii

CHEST'N'LATISSIMUS STRETCH
HANDS ON THE BALL
KNEELING ON THE FLOOR

Primary muscles:
Pectoralis major,
latissimus dorsi, biceps brachii

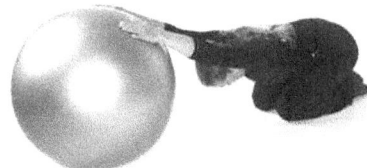

230

Kneeling on the floor behind the ball. One lower leg on the floor, the other foot is on the floor. Working arm relaxed, forearm on the ball. Lean forward towards the ball, while the forearm moves (the ball rolls) in front of the body on the ball. Hold the stretch. Repeat to the other side.	Focus on deep slow breathing. Keep the body in balance and relax all muscles. The stretch can be short, 15-18 seconds for an easy stretch, or longer 30-60 seconds or more for increased flexibility and relaxation.	Different arm/body/leg position.
Kneeling on the floor. The ball is by the side of the body. Same side hand on top of the stability ball, palm down. Keep the torso erect and stable, move the arm backwards along with the stability ball. Hold the stretch. Repeat to the other side.	Keep the torso steady, no rotation, the stretch should be felt in the shoulder muscles. The hand presses down into the ball to keep it from rolling away.	Different arm/body/leg position.
Kneeling on the floor. The ball is by the side of the body. Same side hand on top of the stability ball, palm up. Keep the torso erect and stable, move the arm backwards along with the stability ball. Hold the stretch. Repeat to the other side.	Keep the torso steady, no rotation, the stretch should be felt in the shoulde rmuscles. The hand presses down into the ball to keep it from rolling away.	Different arm/body/leg position.
Kneeling on the floor. The stability ball is in front of the body. Both hands on top of the stability ball. The arms are straight forward, parallel to each other. Push the body downwards and backwards to stretch the back and the chest.	This stretch is normally performed with the hands on the floor. The advantage of using the stability ball is that you may gently roll it for multi-angular stretching.	Different arm/body position.

**CHEST AND LATISSIMUS
STRETCH WITH
BALL ON THE WALL
STANDING ON THE FLOOR**

Primary muscles:
Pectoralis major,
latissimus dorsi

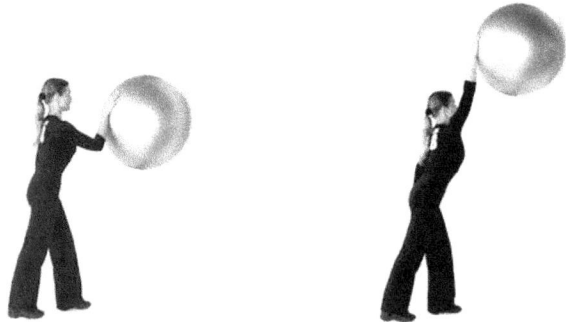

**CHEST STRETCH
WITH BALL ON THE WALL
STANDING ON THE FLOOR**

Primary muscles:
Pectoralis major,
anterior deltoid,
biceps brachii

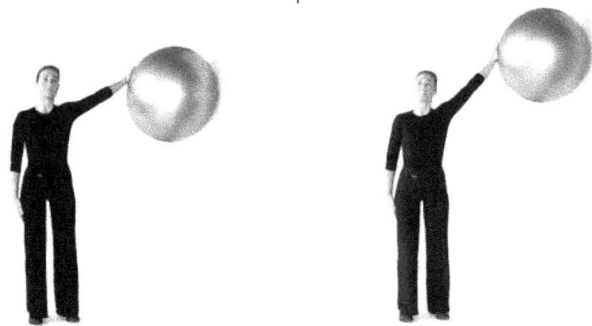

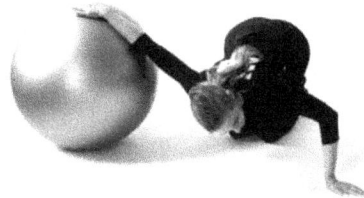

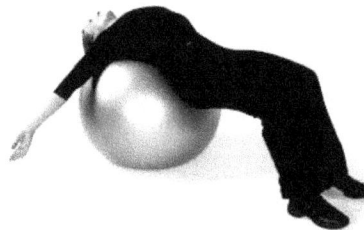

**CHEST STRETCH WITH BALL
KNEELING ON THE FLOOR**

Primary muscles:
Pectoralis major,
anterior deltoid,
biceps brachii

**CHEST STRETCH
SUPINE ON THE BALL**

Primary muscles:
Pectoralis major,
anterior deltoid,
biceps brachii

Standing on the floor by a wall. The body is facing the wall. One hand on the ball, which is held against the wall in front of the body. Move the hand and the ball upwards to stretch the back and the chest. Hold. Change side.	A traditional wall stretch. The advantage of using the stability ball is that you may gently roll it for multi-angular stretching.	Different arm/body/leg position. The ball in different positions.
Standing on the floor by a wall. The side of the body towards the wall. One hand on the ball, which is held against the wall to the side of the body. Move the hand and the ball upwards wall to stretch the chest, shoulder and arm. Roll the ball to stretch the muscles at various angles. Change side.	A traditional wall stretch. The advantage of using the stability ball is that you may gently roll it for multi-angular stretching.	Different arm/body/leg position. The ball in different positions.
Kneeling on the floor. The ball by the side of the body. One hand on top of the ball, other hand to the side and on the floor. Lower the torso gently and rotate the torso away from the ball to increase the chest stretch. Change side.	The advantage of using the stability ball is that you may gently roll it for multi-angular stretching.	Different arm/body/leg position. The ball in different positions.
Supine on the ball. Feet wide apart to stabilize the body and keep the balance. The torso relaxes over the ball, head and neck down to the back. The arms are relaxed and to the side of the ball. The weight of the arms stretches the front of the torso.	The wider the legs, the easier it is to keep the balance. For exercisers who are uncomfortable getting the head too far back: Initially the exercise can be done in an incline, semi-supine position and gradually the body can be moved further backwards.	Different arm/body/leg position.

**CHEST AND LATISSIMUS
STRETCH WITH THE BALL
KNEELING ON THE FLOOR**

Primary muscles:
Pectoralis major, latissimus
dorsi, posterior deltoid

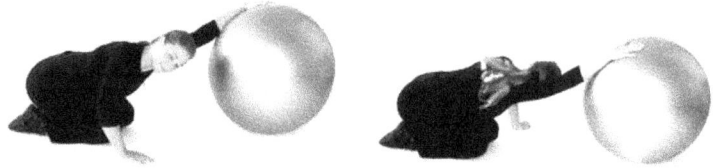

**LATISSIMUS STRETCH
WITH THE BALL
KNEELING ON THE FLOOR**

Primary muscles:
Latissimus dorsi,
posterior deltoid

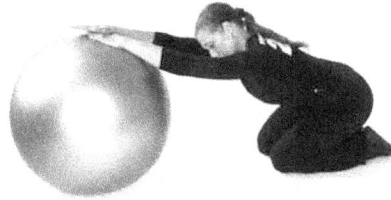

**TORSO STRETCH
WITH THE BALL
KNEELING ON THE FLOOR**

Primary muscles:
Latissimus dorsi,
obliques externus and internus

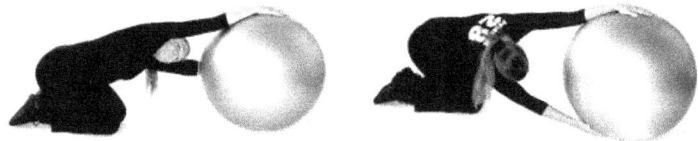

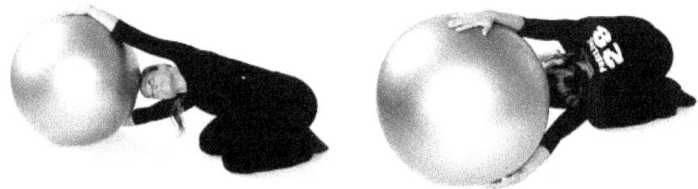

**TORSO STRETCH
HEAD SUPPORTED BY BALL
KNEELING ON THE FLOOR**

Primary muscles:
Latissimus dorsi,
obliques externus and internus

Kneeling on the floor behind the ball. Lower legs on the floor. One hand on top of the ball. Other arm to the side with the hand on the floor. Turn the torso away from the arm on the stability ball. Repeat with the opposite arm on top of the ball.	Make a 'long' spine. Sit heavily on the lower legs, so only the torso rotates to the side.	Different arm/leg position.
Kneeling on the floor behind the ball. Lower legs on the floor. Arms straight forward. Hands on top of the ball. Move the right arm diagonally and put the right hand on top of the left hand to stretch the right side of the torso and the latissimus dorsi. Repeat to the opposite side.	Make a 'long' spine. The torso is kept in line with the legs, only the arms move to the side.	Different body/leg position.
Kneeling on the floor behind the ball. Lower legs on the floor. Arms forward, hands on each side of the stability ball. The head is unsupported. Rotate the stability ball – and the torso – slowly to the side. Rotate to the opposite side.	Focus on deep slow breathing. The stretch can be short, 15-18 seconds for an easy stretch, or longer 30-60 seconds or more for increased flexibility and relaxation.	Different arm/body/leg position.
Kneeling on the floor behind the ball. Lower legs on the floor. Arms forward, hands on each side of the stability ball. The top of the head rests lightly on the ball. Rotate the ball – and the torso – slowly to the side. Rotate to the opposite side.	Focus on deep slow breathing. The stretch can be short, 15-18 seconds for an easy stretch, or longer 30-60 seconds or more for increased flexibility and relaxation.	Different arm/body/leg position.

**CHEST STRETCH
AND SPINAL MOBILITY
SEMI-SUPINE ON THE BALL**

Primary muscles:
Rectus abdominis, obliques,
pectoralis major, latissimus
dorsi

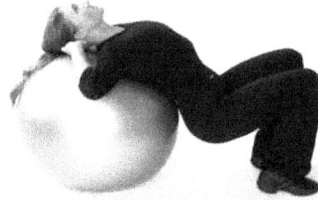

**CHEST STRETCH
AND SPINAL MOBILITY
SUPINE ON THE BALL**

Primary muscles:
Pectoralis major, anterior
deltoid, rectus abdominis,
obliques internus and externus

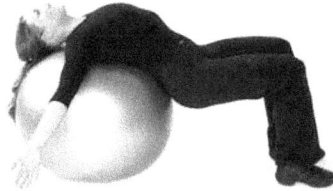

**CHEST STRETCH
AND SPINAL MOBILITY
SUPINE ON THE BALL**

Primary muscles:
Pectoralis major, anterior
deltoid, rectus abdominis,
obliques, latissimus dorsi

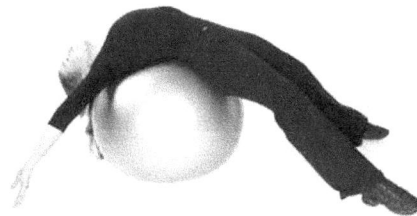

**BACK STRETCH (PLOUGH)
SUPINE ON THE FLOOR**

Primary muscles:
Erector spinae, hamstrings,
gluteus maximus

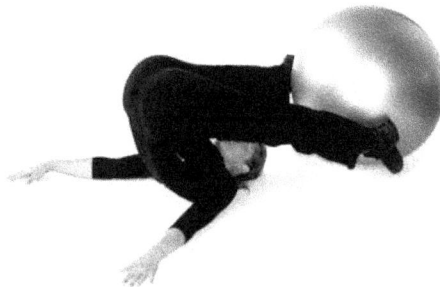

Semi-supine on the ball. Upper back on the ball. Legs bent, lower legs vertical. Feet on the floor shoulder-width apart. Head on the ball, hands behind the head or down by the side.	Focus on deep slow breathing. Keep the body in balance and relax all muscles. The stretch can be short, 15-18 seconds for an easy stretch, or longer 30-60 seconds or more for increased flexibility and relaxation.	Different arm/body/leg position. Different ballsize.
Supine on the ball. Upper and lower back on the ball. Legs bent, lower legs vertical. Feet on the floor, wide apart. Arms to the side. Relax the body, feel 'heavy' and let the weight of the lower body and arms stretch the torso.	Focus on deep slow breathing. Keep the body in balance and relax all muscles. The stretch can be short, 15-18 seconds for an easy stretch, or longer 30-60 seconds or more for increased flexibility and relaxation.	Different arm/body/leg position. Different ballsize and inflation, softer or harder ball.
Supine on the ball. Lower back on top of the ball. Legs relaxed, feet wide apart. Feet on the floor. Arms diagonally back; if possible with the fingertips on the floor. Relax the body, feel 'heavy'; stretch the front of the body and increase spinal mobility.	Focus on deep slow breathing. Keep the body in balance and relax all muscles. The stretch can be short, 15-18 seconds for an easy stretch, or longer 30-60 seconds or more for increased flexibility and relaxation.	Different arm/body/leg position. Different ballsize and inflation, softer or harder ball.
Supine on the floor. Arms at sides. The feet or lower legs hold the ball. Lift the legs and the ball slowly up and over the torso, to put the ball and toes down on the floor behind the head. Hold the position.	For advanced exercisers. Be careful. Support should be on the upper back, not the cervical vertebrae. Perform the stretch slowly and with control. Focus on deep slow breathing.	Different arm/body/leg position. The legs can be bent with the lower legs on the floor on each side of the head.

BACK STRETCH
SITTING ON THE BALL

Primary muscles:
Erector spinae, rhomboids,
trapezius, latissimus dorsi,
gluteus maximus, hamstrings

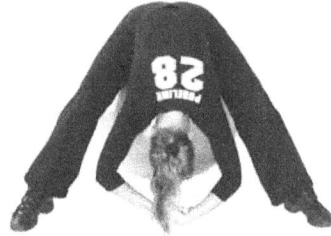

BACK STRETCH
KNEELING ON THE FLOOR
TORSO ON THE BALL

Primary muscles:
Erector spinae, rhomboids,
trapezius, posterior deltoid

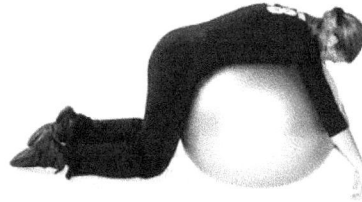

BACK STRETCH
PRONE ON THE BALL

Primary muscles:
Erector spinae, trapezius,
rhomboids, latissimus dorsi

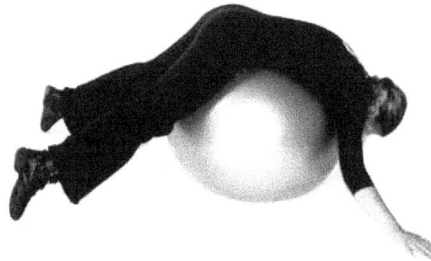

BACK STRETCH
SITTING BEHIND THE BALL

Primary muscles:
Erector spinae, trapezius,
latissimus dorsi, rhomboids,
hamstrings, gluteus maximus,
adductors

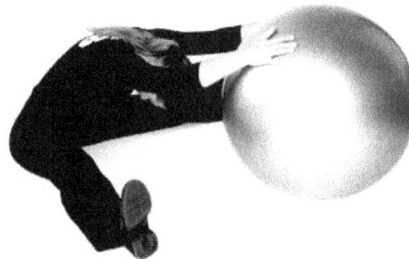

Sitting on the ball. Feet wide apart on the floor. The torso and the arms are completely relaxed and hang down between the legs. Relax the neck and the face. Do not look down on the floor, but towards the ball.	The torso hangs heavily on the ball with the head and neck completely relaxed. Eyes closed. Keep the balance to keep the muscles from contracting. Focus on deep slow breathing, even if it may be a bit difficult in this position.	Different arm/body/leg position. Different ballsize.
Kneeling on the floor behind the ball. Lower legs on the floor. Torso on top of the stability ball. Arms are relaxed and down by the side or slightly in front of the stability ball.	The upper body rests heavily on the ball, completely relaxed. Focus on deep slow breathing, even if it may be difficult with the abdomen resting on the stability ball.	Different arm/body/leg position. Different ballsize.
Prone on the ball. Torso on top of the stability ball with the legs wide apart, toes on the floor. The arms are relaxed and down in front of the stability ball. Hands on the floor.	The body rests heavily on the ball, completely relaxed. Focus on deep slow breathing, even if it may be difficult with the abdomen resting on the stability ball.	Different arm/body/leg position. Different ballsize.
Sitting on the floor behind the ball. Legs wide apart in a straddle position. Hands on top of the ball. Extend the arms forward away from the body and lean the torso forward, so the back and buttocks, and hamstrings and adductors, are stretched.	When the legs are wide, the adductors are stretched.	Different arm/body/leg position.

SIDE STRETCH
WITH BALL IN HANDS
SUPINE ON THE FLOOR

Primary muscles:
Hip and back muscles,
posterior deltoid

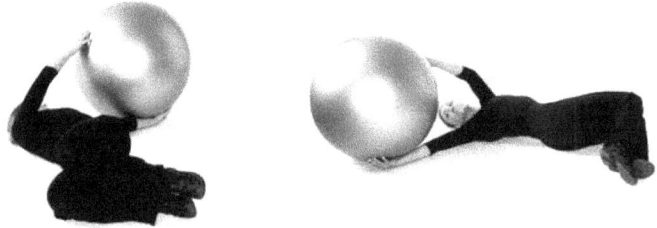

DIAGONAL STRETCH
WITH BALL IN HANDS
SUPINE ON THE FLOOR

Primary muscles:
Pectoralis major, latissimus
dorsi, biceps brachii, deltoids,
hip and back muscles

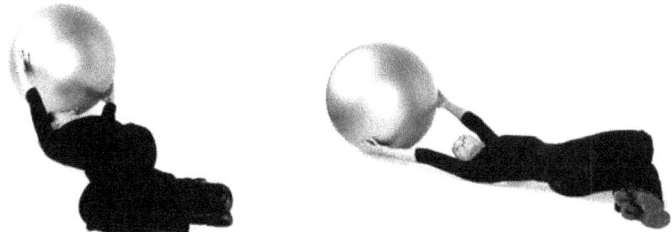

BACK STRETCH, UPRIGHT
HANDS ON THE BALL
KNEELING ON THE FLOOR

Primary muscles:
Trapezius, rhomboids,
erector spinae

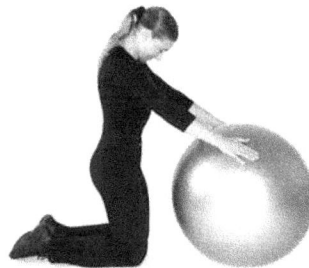

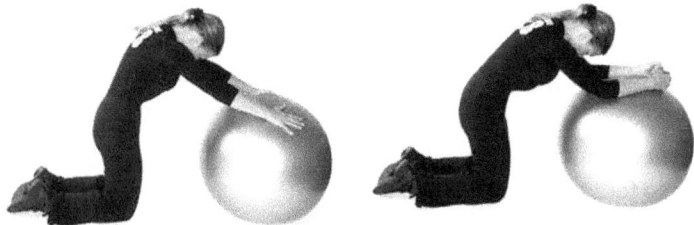

BACK STRETCH
HANDS ON THE BALL
KNEELING BEHIND BALL

Primary muscles:
Trapezius, rhomboids,
erector spinae

Supine on the floor. Feet on the floor. Legs together and bent. Arms vertical with a ball in the hands. Carefully lower the legs to one side. Lower the arms and the ball to the opposite side. Let the ball rest on the floor. Hold and relax in this position. Repeat to the opposite side.	Relax all of the body, let go of any tension; avoid contracting the abdominal and hip muscles. Very relaxing stretch.	Different arm/body/leg position. Hold the stretch or move the ball and legs slowly from side to side.
Supine on the floor. Feet on the floor. Legs together and bent. Arms vertical with a ball in the hands. Carefully lower the legs to one side. Lower the arms and the ball diagonally above the opposite side shoulder. Let the ball rest on the floor. Relax. Repeat opposite side.	Relax all of the body, let go of any tension; avoid contracting the abdominal and hip muscles. Very relaxing diagonal stretch.	Different arm/body/leg position.
Kneeling on the floor behind the ball. Lower legs on the floor, thighs vertical. Torso erect. The hands or forearms are on top of the ball. Round the upper back; push the back upwards and backwards.	Focus on deep slow breathing. The stretch can be short, 15-18 seconds for an easy stretch, or longer 30-60 seconds or more for increased flexibility and relaxation.	Different arm/body/leg position. Different ballsize.
Kneeling on the floor behind the ball. Lower legs on the floor, thighs vertical. The hands or forearms are on the top of the ball. Lean slightly forward at the hips. Round the upper back; push the back upwards and backwards.	Focus on deep slow breathing. Keep the body in balance and relax the muscles. The stretch can be short, 15-18 seconds for an easy stretch, or longer 30-60 seconds or more for increased flexibility and relaxation.	Different arm/body/leg position. Different ballsize.

BACK STRETCH
HANDS ON THE BALL
STANDING ON THE FLOOR

Primary muscles:
Rhomboids,
trapezius, erector spinae

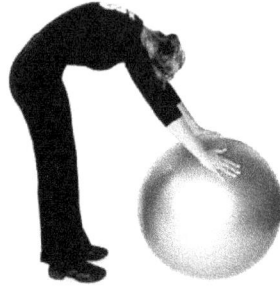

BACK STRETCH
FOREARMS ON THE BALL
STANDING ON THE FLOOR

Primary muscles:
Erector spinae, rhomboids,
trapezius

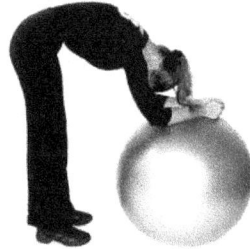

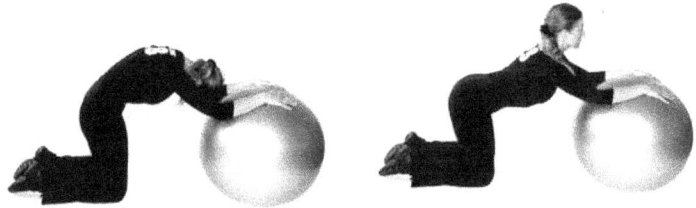

CAT-CAMEL
FOREARMS ON THE BALL
KNEELING ON THE FLOOR

Primary muscles:
Erector spinae, rhomboids,
trapezius

HIP STRETCH TO THE SIDE
HANDS ON THE BALL
KNEELING ON THE FLOOR

Primary muscles:
Hip muscles, obliques externus
and internus, latissimus dorsi

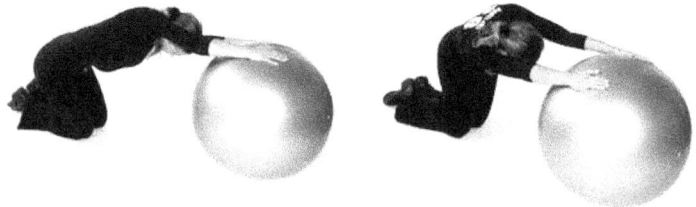

Standing behind the ball. Feet hip-width apart. Torso forward. Hands on top of the ball. Round the back upwards to stretch the muscles on the backside of the body. Focus on the muscles between the shoulder blades.	Focus on deep slow breathing. You may relax the knees slightly, if the stretch is too hard on the hamstrings.	Different arm/body/leg position. Different ballsize.
Standing behind the ball. Feet hip-width apart. Torso forward. Forearms on top of the ball. Round the back to stretch the muscles on the backside of the body. Focus on the back extensors and the lower back.	Focus on deep slow breathing. You can relax the knees slightly, if the stretch is too hard on the hamstrings.	Different arm/body/leg position. Different ballsize.
Kneeling behind the ball. Torso forward. Forearms on top of the ball. Round the back and look to the stomach. Relax and arch the back a little, look forward. Breathe deeply.	Excellent mobility exercise for the spine. You can work on your breathing along with the movement: Inhale when sagging the back, exhale when rounding the back. Focus on deep slow breathing.	Different arm/body/leg position. Different ballsize.
Kneeling behind the ball. Lower legs on the floor. Torso forward. Forearms on top of the ball. Move the hips out to one side, feel the stretch along the side of the body. Repeat to the other side.	Mobility exercise. Focus on deep slow breathing. Make the movement smaller, tail wagging, move the hips side to side, for lumbar spine mobility.	Different arm/body/leg position.

SIDE STRETCH WITH BALL
OPPOSITE ARM ON BALL
SITTING ON THE FLOOR

Primary muscles:
Latissimus dorsi,
obliques externus and
internus, adductors

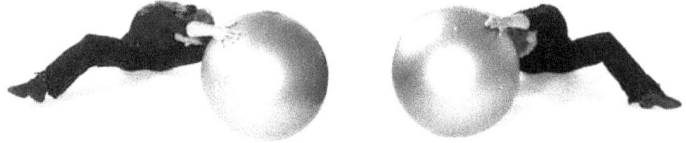

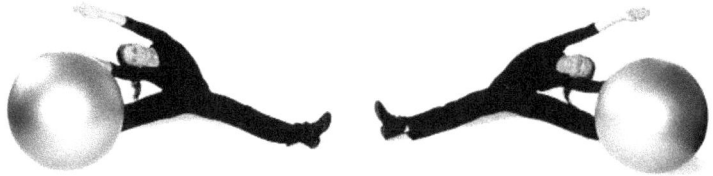

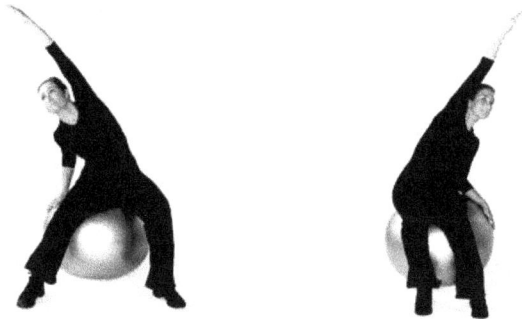

SIDE STRETCH WITH BALL
SAME SIDE ARM ON BALL
SITTING ON THE FLOOR

Primary muscles:
Latissimus dorsi,
obliques externus and
internus, adductors

SIDE STRETCH
SITTING ON THE BALL

Primary muscles:
Latissimus dorsi,
obliques externus and internus

SIDE STRETCH, DIAGONAL,
SITTING ON THE BALL

Primary muscles:
Latissimus dorsi,
erector spinae,
obliques externus and internus

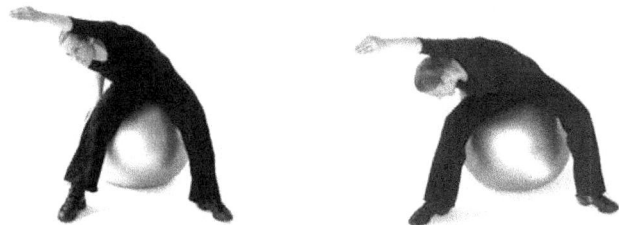

Sitting on the floor behind the ball. The legs are bent and wide apart in straddle position. Right arm on top of the ball. Roll the ball to the left foot to stretch the right side. Left arm relaxed by the side of the body or left hand on the right elbow. Repeat to the other side.	Focus on deep slow breathing. Keep the body in balance and relax all muscles. The stretch can be short, 15-18 seconds for an easy stretch, or longer 30-60 seconds or more for increased flexibility and relaxation.	Different arm/body/leg position. Legs can be bent or straight.
Sitting on the floor behind the ball. The legs are straight and wide apart in straddle position. Right arm on top of the ball. Roll the ball to the right foot to stretch the left side. The left arm is overhead, hand to the right to increase the stretch. Repeat to the other side.	For intermediate to advanced exercisers. Requires some adductor and hamstring flexibility. Focus on deep slow breathing. Keep the body in balance and relax all muscles.	Different arm/body/leg position. Legs can be straight or bent.
Sitting on the ball. Feet on the floor hip-width apart. Right hand support on the ball, the left arm is reaching over the head to the right to increase the stretch. Hold. Repeat to the other side.	Focus on deep slow breathing. Keep the body in balance and relax all muscles. The stretch can be short, 15-18 seconds for an easy stretch, or longer 30-60 seconds or more for increased flexibility and relaxation.	Different arm/body/leg position. You can move the hips and the arm in different angles.
Sitting on the ball. Feet on the floor hip-width apart. Right hand support on the ball, the left arm is reaching up. Rotate the torso and reach the left arm diagonally towards the opposite leg to increase the back (latissimus dorsi) stretch. Repeat to the other side.	Focus on deep slow breathing. Keep the body in balance and relax all muscles. The stretch can be short, 15-18 seconds for an easy stretch, or longer 30-60 seconds or more for increased flexibility and relaxation.	Different arm/body/leg position. You can move the hips and the arm in different angles. Eg. the arm can be in the horizontal plane or down towards the opposite foot.

**SIDE STRETCH
SIDELYING ON THE BALL
BOTTOM LEG KNEELING**

Primary muscles:
Latissimus dorsi,
obliques externus and internus

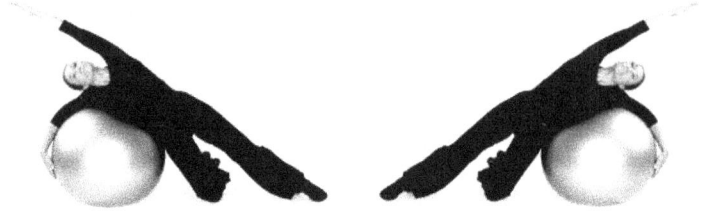

**SIDE STRETCH
STRAIGHT LEGS
SIDELYING ON THE BALL**

Primary muscles:
Latissimus dorsi,
obliques,
gluteus medius and minimus

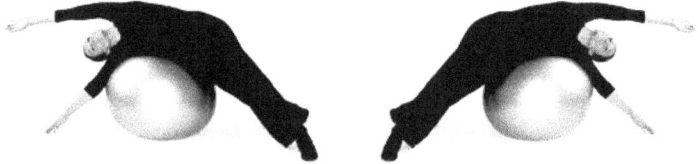

**HIP AND LOWER BACK
STRETCH
LEGS AROUND THE BALL
SUPINE ON THE FLOOR**

Primary muscles:
Gluteus maximus,
obliques externus and internus

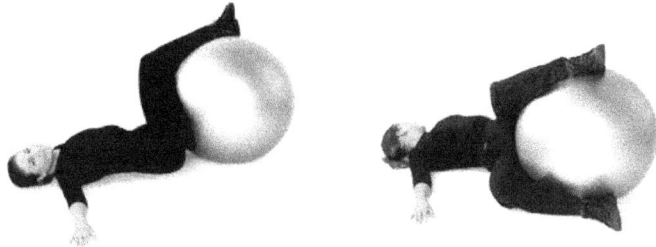

**TORSO STRETCH
SITTING ON THE BALL**

Primary muscles:
Pectoralis major, deltoids
anterior (photo 1), rhomboids,
latissimus dorsi, trapezius,
posterior deltoid (photo 2)

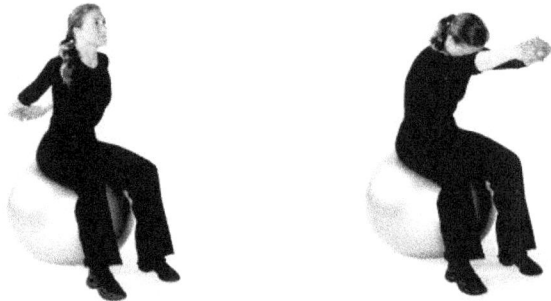

Kneeling on the floor by the side of the ball. Bottom leg bent, lower leg on the floor. Top leg straight, the foot is on the floor, and in line with the torso. Bottom hand on the ball. Top arm reaching overhead. Lean the body over the ball to stretch the side. Repeat to the other side.	Focus on deep slow breathing. The stretch can be short, 15-18 seconds for an easy stretch, or longer 30-60 seconds or more for increased flexibility and relaxation.	Different arm/body/leg position. Different ballsize.
Sidelying on the ball. Legs straight and staggered on the floor to keep the body in balance. Bottom hand is down on the floor. Top arm is reaching over the head to increase the stretch. Repeat to the other side.	Focus on deep slow breathing. Relax all muscles. The stretch can be short, 15-18 seconds for an easy stretch, or longer 30-60 seconds or more for increased flexibility and relaxation.	Different arm/body/leg position. Different ballsize.
Supine on the floor. Lower legs on top of the ball, a little apart to control the ball. Hamstrings touch the ball. Arms to the side. Contract the obliques slightly to control the movement and slowly rotate the ball and legs to the side to stretch the hips and low back. Hold. Repeat to the other side.	Focus on deep slow breathing. The stretch can be short, 15-18 seconds for an easy stretch, or longer 30-60 seconds or more for increased flexibility and relaxation.	Different arm/body/leg position.
Sitting on the ball. Feet on the floor hip-width apart. Hands together. Move the arms forward and up and backward to stretch the torso, the shoulders and arms at different angles.	Focus on deep slow breathing. Keep the body in balance. The stretch can be short, 15-18 seconds for an easy stretch, or longer 30-60 seconds or more for increased flexibility.	Different arm/body/leg position.

**HIP AND BUTTOCK STRETCH
SUPINE ON THE FLOOR**

Primary muscles:
Gluteus maximus, medius and
minimus, piriformis

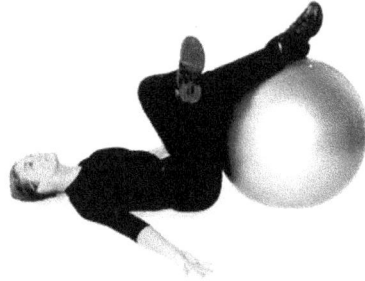

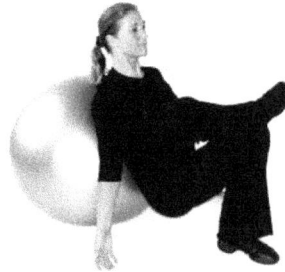

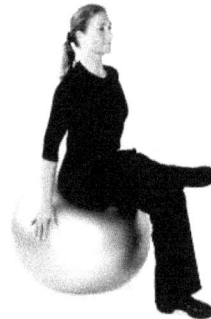

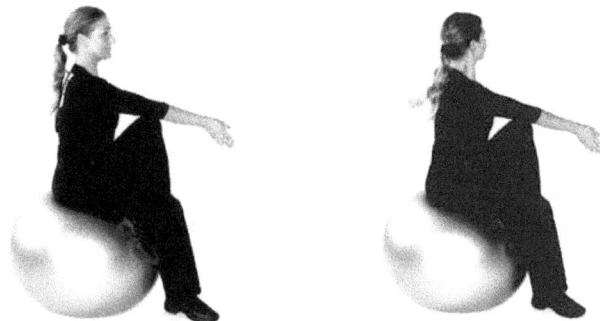

**HIP AND BUTTOCK STRETCH
SEMI-SUPINE ON THE BALL**

Primary muscles:
Gluteus maximus, medius and
minimus, piriformis

**HIP AND BUTTOCK STRETCH
SITTING ON THE BALL**

Primary muscles:
Gluteus maximus, medius and
minimus, piriformis

**HIP AND BUTTOCK STRETCH
SITTING ON THE BALL
ONE FOOT ON THE BALL**

Primary muscles:
Gluteus maximus, medius and
minimus, piriformis

Supine on the floor. The arms are on the floor. The left lower leg is on top of the ball. The right leg is bent and crossed over the left with the foot resting on the left thigh. Rotate the right leg to the side, knee out. Repeat with the opposite leg.	Focus on deep slow breathing. Relax all muscles. Roll the ball side to side for multi-angular stretching. The stretch can be short, 15-18 seconds for an easy stretch, or longer 30-60 seconds or more for increased flexibility.	Different arm/body/leg position. Turn the palms upwards to open and relax the shoulders.
Semi-supine on the ball. The back is leaning on the ball, the head and neck and the buttocks are off the ball. The arms are down at sides, Both legs are bent. Left foot on the floor, lower leg vertical. Right leg crossed over the left and rotated to the side. Repeat with the opposite leg.	Focus on deep slow breathing. Find the balance; be careful, that the ball does not roll away from you, so you fall. The stretch can be short, 15-18 seconds for an easy stretch, or longer 30-60 seconds or more for increased flexibility.	Different arm/body/leg position.
Sitting on the ball. Arms at sides. Hands on the ball. Both legs are bent. Left foot on the floor, lower leg vertical. Right leg crossed over the left. Rotate the right leg to the side, knee out. Repeat with the opposite leg.	For intermediate to advanced exercisers. Keep the balance. Focus on deep slow breathing. The stretch can be short, 15-18 seconds for an easy stretch, or longer 30-60 seconds for increased flexibility.	Different arm/body/leg position. Lean the torso forward to stretch the hip in different angles.
Sitting on the ball. Both legs are bent. Right foot on the floor, lower leg vertical. Left leg crossed over the right, the foot is on the ball by the opposite knee. Rotate the torso and put the right arm on the outside of the left leg to increase the stretch. Repeat with the opposite leg.	Focus on deep slow breathing. Keep the balance. The stretch can be short, 15-18 seconds for an easy stretch, or longer 30-60 seconds or more for increased flexibility.	Different arm/body/leg position.

**HIP AND BUTTOCK STRETCH,
LUNGE POSITION
ON THE FLOOR
SUPPORT ON THE BALL**

Primary muscles:
Iliopsoas and rectus femoris,
gluteus maximus

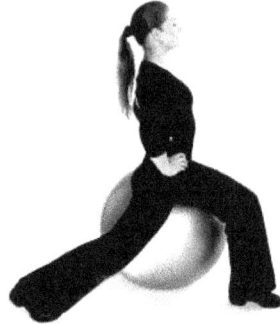

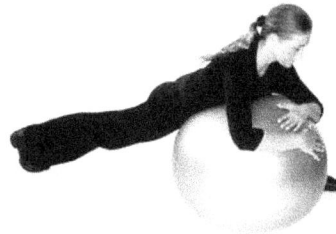

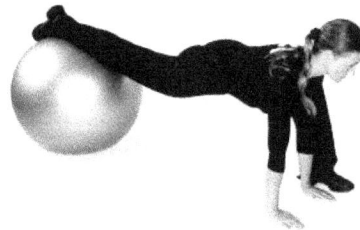

**HIP AND BUTTOCK STRETCH,
LUNGE POSITION
ON THE FLOOR
AB SUPPORTED ON BALL**

Primary muscles:
Iliopsoas and rectus femoris,
gluteus maximus

**HIP FLEXOR STRETCH
LUNGE POSITION
FRONT FOOT ON THE FLOOR
BACK LEG ON THE BALL**

Primary muscles:
Iliopsoas and rectus femoris,
gluteus maximus

**HIP FLEXOR STRETCH
PRONE ON THE BALL
IN BALANCE PLANK**

Primary muscles:
Iliopsoas and rectus femoris

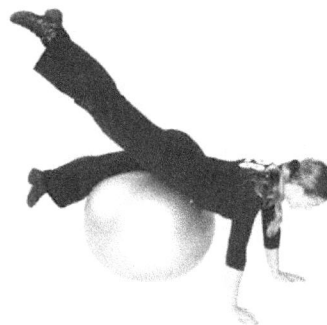

Standing on the floor. Lunge position by the side of the ball. Ball by the side of the front leg. Roll the ball under the front leg hamstrings and buttock. Sit on the ball to go deeper into the stretch – you are supported by the stability ball. Repeat with the opposite leg.	Start in a perfect, stable, stationary lunge position, before placing the ball and sitting into the stretch. Both legs are bent. Feet and knees are aligned, no rotation of the knees. Front foot is firmly on the floor, back leg heel is lifted.	Different arm/body/leg position. Range of motion, depth of the lunge, may vary.
Standing on the floor. Deep lunge position. The stability ball is by the inside of the front leg. The torso is leaning forward and resting on the stability ball. The arms hug the ball. Repeat with the opposite leg.	For intermediate to advanced exercisers. Go down into a deep lunge. Feet and knees are aligned, no rotation of the knees. Front foot is firmly on the floor, back leg heel is lifted.	Different arm/body/leg position. Range of motion, depth of the lunge, may vary.
Standing on the floor. Deep lunge. Front foot on the floor, knee bent 90 degrees. Lower leg vertical. Torso forward, shoulders over the hands. Hands on the floor by the inside of the leg. Back leg straight, foot and lower leg is on top of the ball. Repeat with the opposite leg.	For advanced exercisers. Focus on deep slow breathing.	Different arm/body/leg position. Range of motion, depth of the lunge, may vary.
Plank position. Hips on the stability ball. Hands on the floor. Lift one leg up into hip extension to actively stretch the hip flexors of that leg. Hold. Repeat with the opposite leg.	For intermediate exercisers. An active stretch: The buttocks contract to lift the leg and stretch the hip flexor. Focus on deep slow breathing.	Different arm/body/leg position. On the hips or the thighs.

HIP AND GLUTE STRETCH
ARMS ON THE BALL
SITTING ON THE FLOOR

Primary muscles:
Gluteus maximus, piriformis,
iliopsoas and rectus femoris

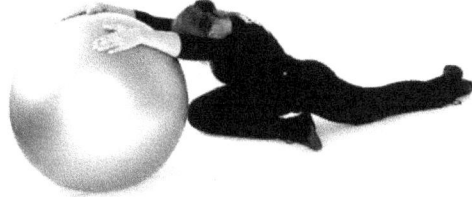

HIP AND GLUTE STRETCH
ONE ARM ON THE BALL
SITTING ON THE FLOOR

Primary muscles:
Iliopsoas, quadriceps,
gluteus maximus

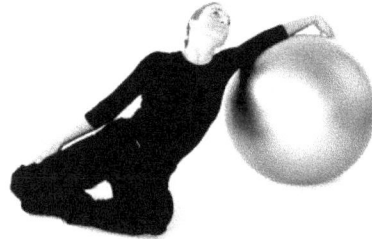

HIP AND QUAD STRETCH
SUPPORTING ON THE BALL
KNEELING ON THE FLOOR

Primary muscles:
Iliopsoas, quadriceps

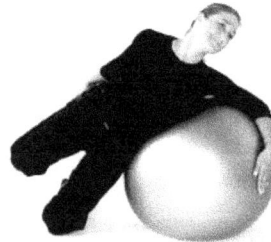

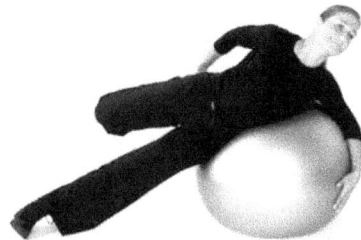

HIP AND QUAD STRETCH
SIDELYING ON THE BALL

Primary muscles:
Iliopsoas, quadriceps

Sitting on the floor. One leg bent and externally rotated, knee out to the side, foot in front of the body. Other leg is straight and extended straight back on the floor. Torso forward. Hands on top of the ball. Relax. Repeat with the opposite leg.	Relax completely.	Different arm/body/leg position. Range of motion, depth of the lunge, may vary.
Sitting on the floor. Ball by the side of the body. Arm on top of the ball. Both legs bent 90 degrees or more. One leg is in front of the body, the other behind. You sit on the front leg and bend the back leg a little more to increase the quad and hip flexor stretch. Repeat opposite leg.	For intermediate to advanced exercisers with flexible hip muscles. Avoid rotation of the knees. Check that knees and feet are aligned.	Different arm/body/leg position.
Kneeling on the floor. Ball by the side of the body. Rest the torso on the ball, stabilize with the arm. Bottom lower leg on the floor. Bend the top leg, take hold of the ankle with the hand, and stretch the quad and hip flexor. Top leg is behind the bottom leg. Repeat with the opposite leg.	Keep the balance. Working leg is in line with the torso, no abduction or rotation at the hip. Hold the ankle, not the toes.	Different arm/body/leg position.
Sidelying on the ball. Arm around the ball to stabilize. Bottom leg straight, side of the foot on the floor. Bend the top leg, take hold of the ankle with the hand, and stretch the quad and hip flexor. Top leg is behind the bottom leg. Repeat with the opposite leg.	Keep the balance. Working leg is in line with the torso, no abduction or rotation at the hip (on this photo there is a slight abduction). Hold the ankle, not the toes.	Different arm/body/leg position.

**QUAD STRETCH
ONE LEG ON THE BALL
KNEELING ON THE FLOOR**

Primary muscles:
Quadriceps, iliopsoas

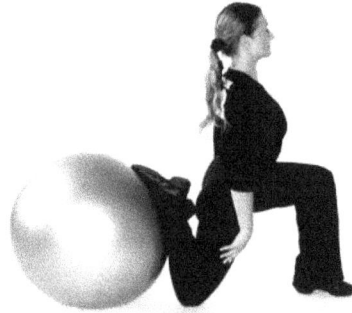

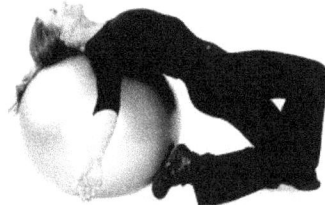

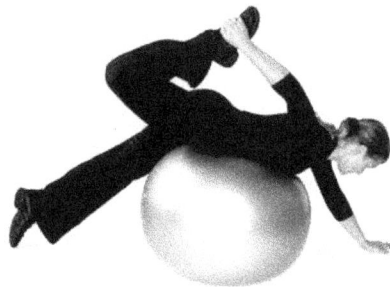

**QUAD AND TIBIALIS STRETCH
ONE LEG ON THE BALL
KNEELING ON THE FLOOR**

Primary muscles:
Quadriceps, iliopsoas,
tibialis anterior

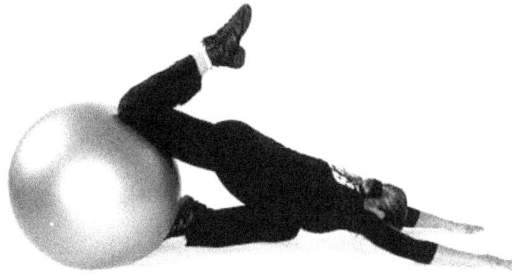

**QUAD STRETCH
BRIDGE POSITION
ON THE BALL**

Primary muscles:
Quadriceps, iliopsoas

**QUAD STRETCH
PRONE ON THE BALL**

Primary muscles:
Quadriceps, iliopsoas

Kneeling on the floor in front of the ball. Front foot on the floor, knee bent 90 degrees. Back leg bent, lower leg and ankle against the ball, the knee (just above the kneecap) is on the floor. Torso is erect, so the hip is stretched. Arm position is optional. Repeat with the opposite leg.	For intermediate exercisers to advanced exercisers. Avoid supporting your bodyweight directly on the kneecap – as this is very uncomfortable – and position the knee on a soft mat.	Different arm/body/leg position.
On all fours on the floor. One lower leg on the floor. Other leg on top of the ball. Bend the top leg. Plantarflex the ankle to stretch the quad and tibialis. At the same time slide the torso and arms forward and down. Repeat with the opposite leg.	For intermediate to advanced exercisers. An active tibialis stretch, so the leg may cramp; relax, shake the leg, and try again. May be uncomfortable if you have knee problems. If so, use another stretch.	Different arm/body/leg position.
Bridge position on the ball. Contract the buttocks slightly to hold the position. Upper body on the stability ball. Left foot in front firmly on the floor, knee bent 90 degrees. Right leg bent, lower leg close to the floor behind the right leg. Repeat with the opposite leg.	Focus on deep slow breathing. Keep the buttocks contracted. The stretch can be short, 15-18 seconds for an easy stretch, or longer 30-60 seconds or more for increased flexibility and relaxation.	Different arm/body/leg position. Different ball size.
Prone on the ball. One hand on the floor in front of the stability ball. The other hand holds the ankle of the same side leg. The leg is bent and lifted to stretch the quad and hip flexor. The other leg is straight with toes on the floor. Repeat with the opposite leg.	For intermediate and advanced exercisers. Keep the neck in neutral position. The legs are kept as close to each other (the midline of the body) as possible.	Different arm/body/leg position. Different ballsize.

**HAMSTRING STRETCH
ONE LEG BENT,
ONE LEG STRAIGHT
SITTING ON THE BALL**

Primary muscles:
Gluteus maximus, hamstring

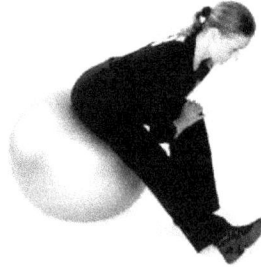

**HAMSTRING STRETCH
LEGS STRAIGHT
SITTING ON THE BALL**

Primary muscles:
Gluteus maximus, hamstrings

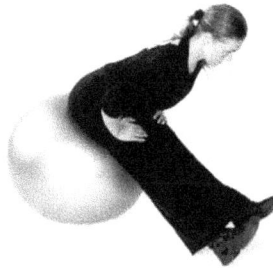

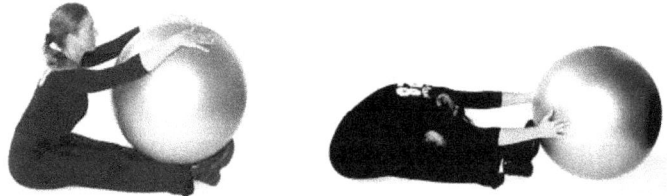

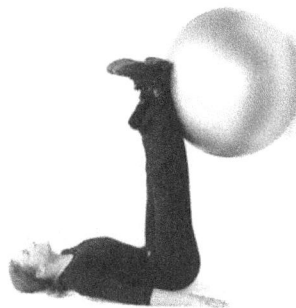

**HAMSTRING STRETCH
SITTING ON THE FLOOR**

Primary muscles:
Gluteus maximus, hamstrings

**HAMSTRING STRETCH
SUPINE, FEET ON THE BALL
BALL AGAINST ON THE WALL**

Primary muscles:
Gluteus maximus, hamstrings

Sitting on the ball. Feet are on the floor. One leg bent, other leg straight, heel on the floor. The hands are on the thigh(s). Push the buttocks back and lean slightly forward with the torso to increase the hamstring stretch of the straight leg. Repeat with the opposite leg.	Legs can be wider apart, so it is easier to keep the balance, but then position the torso over the working leg, not between the two legs. Be careful not to press the hands down on the straight leg; avoid hyperextending the knee.	Different arm/body/leg position. Hands on the bent leg or on the ball.
Sitting on the ball. The feet, heels, are on the floor. Both legs straight, knees relaxed. Hands on the thighs. Push the buttocks back and lean slightly forward with the torso to increase the hamstring stretch.	Focus on deep slow breathing. The stretch can be short, 15-18 seconds for an easy stretch, or longer 30-60 seconds or more for increased flexibility.	Different arm/body/leg position.
Sitting on the floor. Legs straight forward in front of the body. Back straight. Hands on the ball on the legs (left photo), on the toes or in front of the feet (right photo), for an increased stretch. Lean forward at the hips to increase the stretch. Repeat with the opposite leg.	Focus on deep slow breathing. Relax all muscles. The stretch can be short, 15-18 seconds for an easy stretch, or longer 30-60 seconds or more for increased flexibility.	Different arm/body/leg position.
Supine on the floor by a wall. Arms on the floor. Legs bent, feet against the ball. Walk the feet on the ball, rolling it up to a higher position: Legs vertical, buttocks and legs close to wall. The lower legs are on the ball held against the wall.	A traditional wall stretch. The advantage of using the stability ball, is that you may gently roll the ball for some multi-angular stretching.	Different arm/body/leg position.

HAMSTRING STRETCH
ONE LEG ON THE BALL
SUPINE ON THE FLOOR

Primary muscles:
Gluteus maximus, hamstrings

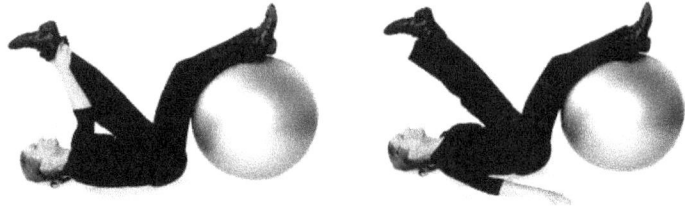

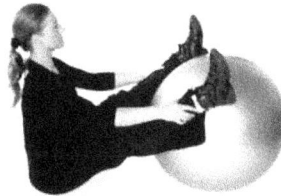

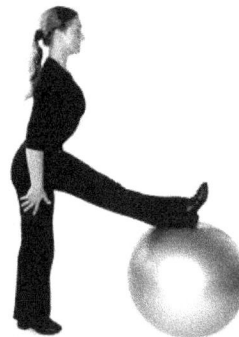

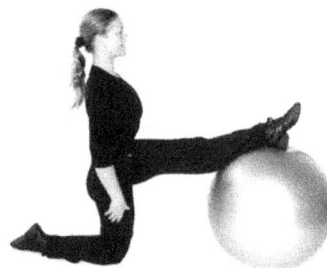

HAMSTRING STRETCH
BOTH LEGS ON THE BALL
SITTING ON THE FLOOR

Primary muscles:
Gluteus maximus, hamstrings

HAMSTRING STRETCH
ONE LEG ON THE BALL
STANDING ON THE FLOOR

Primary muscles:
Gluteus maximus, hamstrings

HAMSTRING STRETCH
ONE LEG ON THE BALL
KNEELING ON THE FLOOR

Primary muscles:
Gluteus maximus, hamstrings

Supine on the floor. One lower leg on the stability ball. Other leg straight, up and off the ball. Hold the leg with the hands. Pull gently at the leg to bring it closer to the torso. Keep the leg straight. Hold the stretch. Repeat with the opposite leg.	Passive stretch: The arms are holding the leg. Active stretch: Let go of the arms and contract the hip flexor to bring the leg closer to the torso.	Different arm/body/leg position. Active or passive stretch. The knee of the working leg can be bent (focus on the buttocks) or straight (focus on the hamstrings).
Sitting on the floor. Feet on top of the ball, hip- or shoulder-width apart. The hands are on the legs or on the ball. Start in a V-sit position with bent legs and then slowly stretch the legs. Hold the stretch.	For advanced exercisers. Requires some flexibility and balance.	Different arm/body/leg position. The same type of stretch can be performed sitting on the stability ball with the feet on the floor.
Standing on the floor behind the ball. Arms at sides. One foot on the floor. The other leg is straight and the heel is on top of the ball. Lean slightly forward at the hips, push the buttocks back to increase the stretch. Repeat with the opposite leg.	For intermediate exercisers. Requires some balance. Keep the balance. Focus on deep slow breathing.	Different arm/body/leg position. The knee of the working leg can be bent (focus on the buttocks) or straight (focus on the hamstrings).
Kneeling on the floor behind the ball. Arms at sides. One lower leg on the floor. The other leg is straight and the lower leg is on top of the ball. Lean slightly forward at the hips to increase the stretch. Repeat with the opposite leg.	For intermediate to advanced exercisers. Requires some flexibility and balance. Focus on deep slow breathing. Keep the balance.	Different arm/body/leg position. The knee of the working leg can be bent (focus on the buttocks) or straight (focus on the hamstrings).

ADDUCTOR STRETCH
FOREARMS ON THE BALL
STANDING ON THE FLOOR

Primary muscles:
Adductors

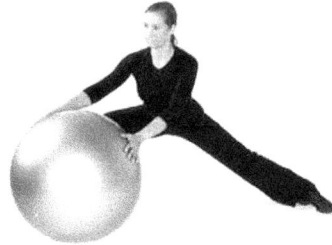

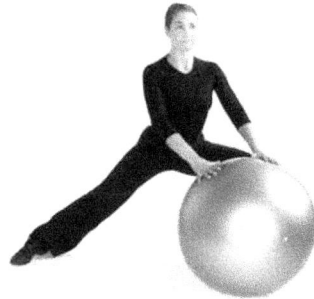

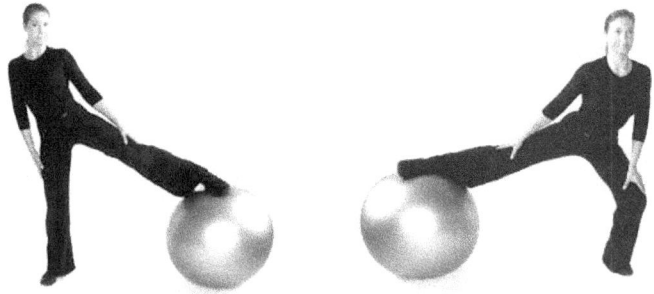

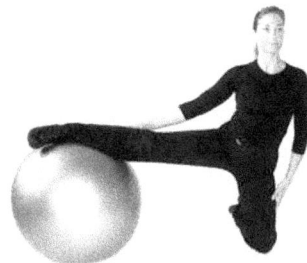

ADDUCTOR STRETCH
HANDS ON THE BALL
STANDING ON THE FLOOR

Primary muscles:
Adductors

ADDUCTOR STRETCH
ONE LEG ON THE BALL
STANDING ON THE FLOOR

Primary muscles:
Adductors

ADDUCTOR STRETCH
ONE LEG ON THE BALL
KNEELING ON THE FLOOR

Primary muscles:
Adductors

Standing on the floor behind the ball. Feet wide apart. One leg is bent, the other is straight – side lunge position. Torso forward, forearms on the ball (not hands as in photo). The foot and knee of the stretch leg points forward. Repeat with the opposite leg.	Focus on deep slow breathing. The stretch can be short, 15-18 seconds for an easy stretch, or longer 30-60 seconds for increased flexibility.	Different arm/body/leg position.
Standing on the floor behind the ball. Torso erect. Hands on the ball. Legs wide apart in lunge position: One leg is bent, the other leg is straight. Repeat with the opposite leg.	Focus on deep slow breathing. The stretch can be short, 15-18 seconds for an easy stretch, or longer 30-60 seconds for increased flexibility.	Different arm/body/leg position.
Standing on the floor by the side of the ball. Supporting leg on the floor is either straight or bent, The other leg is straight and lifted to the side up on top of the stability ball. Torso erect. Arms at sides or on thighs. Repeat with the opposite leg.	For intermediate exercisers. Focus on deep slow breathing. Keep the balance. Do not put too much pressure on the knees, as this may feel uncomfortable. Reduce the range of motion if needed.	Different arm/body/leg position. Perform standing or kneeling.
Kneeling on the floor by the side of the ball. Torso erect. The hands support on the legs. Supporting leg, lower leg is on the floor. The other leg is straight and lifted to the side, on top of the stability ball. Repeat with the opposite leg.	For intermediate exercisers. Keep the balance. May be uncomfortable for the knees; remember to relax the top knee and rest the lower leg on a mat.	Different arm/body/leg position.

ADDUCTOR STRETCH
SITTING ON THE BALL

Primary muscles:
Adductors

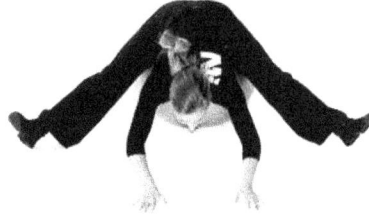

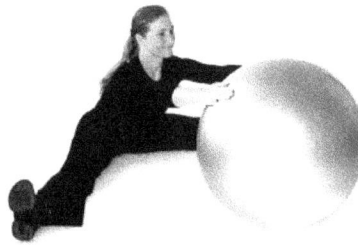

ADDUCTOR STRETCH
HANDS ON THE BALL IN
FRONT OF THE BODY
SITTING ON THE FLOOR

Primary muscles:
Adductors

ABDUCTOR STRETCH
BALL IN HANDS
STANDING ON THE FLOOR

Primary muscles:
Gluteus medius,
gluteus minimus

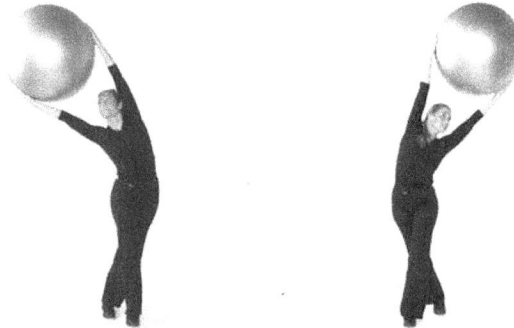

CALF STRETCH
HANDS ON THE BALL
STANDING ON THE FLOOR

Primary muscles:
Gastrocnemeus, soleus

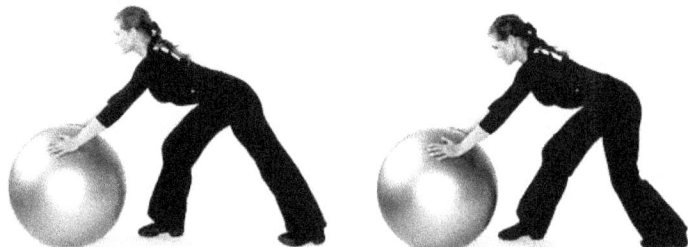

Sitting on the ball. Feet on the floor. Legs straight and in a wide straddle position. Lean forward at the hips and put the hands on the floor. Relax the torso and arms. The torso is between the legs.	Focus on deep slow breathing. Keep the balance. The stretch can be short, 15-18 seconds for an easy stretch, or longer 30-60 seconds for increased flexibility.	Different arm/body/leg position. Keep the back straight, focus on the adductor stretch, or relax and round the back, focus on stretching the back and the buttocks.
Sitting on the floor behind the ball. Legs wide, straddle position. The ball is between the legs. Hands on top of the ball. The back is straight. Slowly roll the stability ball away from the body, so the torso is leaning forward at the hips to stretch the adductors.	For intermediate exercisers. Requires some adductor and hamstring flexibility. Focus on deep slow breathing. The stretch can be short, 15-18 seconds for an easy stretch, or longer 30-60 seconds for increased flexibility.	Different arm/body/leg position. Keep the back straight, focus on the adductor stretch, or relax and round the back, focus on stretching the back and the buttocks.
Standing on the floor. Legs are almost straight. Right leg is crossed behind the left. Move the right hip out to the right. Arms are overhead with the ball in the hands. The torso, arms and balls are leaning slightly to the left. Contract the core. Repeat to the other side.	Keep the balance. Focus on deep slow breathing. The stretch can be short, 15-18 seconds for an easy stretch, or longer 30-60 seconds for increased flexibility.	Different arm/body/leg position.
Standing behind the ball. Hands on the ball. Legs staggered. Front leg is bent. Back leg is straight and heel is on the floor. Stretch the calf muscles. Bend the back leg, but keep the heel on the floor. Stretch. Repeat with the opposite leg.	Focus on deep slow breathing. Keep the balance.	Different arm/body/leg position. The back leg can be straight or bent, focus on gastrocnemeus or soleus.

CALF STRETCH
PLANK POSITION
FOREARMS ON THE BALL

Primary muscles:
Gastrocnemeus, soleus

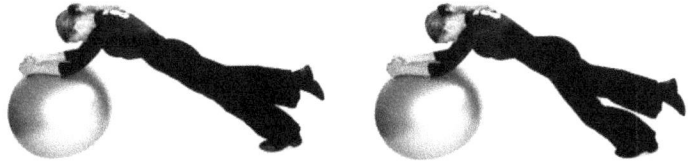

CALF STRETCH
HANDS ON THE BALL
STANDING ON THE FLOOR

Primary muscles:
Gastrocnemeus, soleus,
gluteus maximus, hamstrings

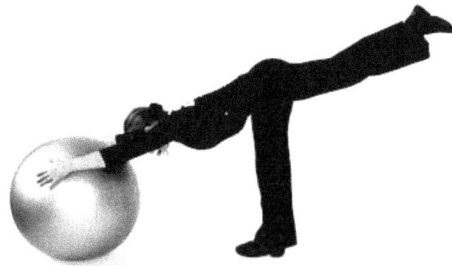

CALF STRETCH
KNEELING ON THE FLOOR

Primary muscles:
Soleus, gastrocnemeus

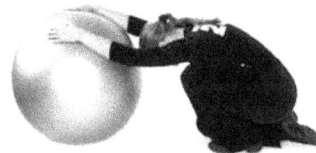

TIBIALIS STRETCH
KNEELING ON THE FLOOR

Primary muscles:
Tibialis anterior

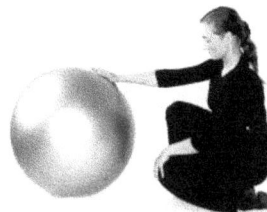

Plank position. Forearms on the ball. Core muscles contract to stabilize the body. Support on one leg, heel close to the floor to stretch the calf muscles. Leg straight or bent. The other leg is lifted slightly off the floor. Hold. Repeat with the opposite leg.	For advanced exercisers. Focus on deep slow breathing. Keep the balance.	Different arm/body/leg position. The supporting leg can be straight or bent, focus on gastrocnemeus or soleus.
Standing on the floor. Hands on the ball. One foot on the floor. Other leg is lifted into a sagittal split position if possible. Roll the ball forward, so the body leans forward, in line with the lifted leg. Keep the heel of the supporting leg on the floor. Repeat with the opposite leg.	For advanced exercisers. Focus on deep slow breathing. Keep the balance. The stretch can be short, 15-18 seconds for an easy stretch, or longer 30-60 seconds, for increased flexibility.	Different arm/body/leg position. The supporting leg can be straight or bent, focus on gastrocnemeus or soleus.
Kneeling on the floor. One lower leg on the floor, other leg bent with the foot on the floor. Arms around the ball. Move the leg on the floor forward, so the knee is in front of the supporting foot. Move the torso forward on the thigh to press the leg down. Repeat with the opposite leg.	Focus on deep slow breathing. Keep the heel on the floor. Some exercisers do not feel the stretch right away. Then do another stretch. Or vary the position a little; heel all the way down, bottom knee forward or torso forward.	Different arm/body/leg position.
Kneeling on the floor. Right foot on the floor, left lower leg, shin, on the floor. Torso erect. Right hand on the ball. The left hand lifts the left knee off the floor, so the front of the left lower leg is stretched. Bodyweight over the supporting leg. Repeat with the opposite leg.	Focus on deep slow breathing. Some exercisers do not feel the stretch right away. Then do another stretch. Or if vary the position a little; move the stretch leg or the body.	Different arm/body/leg position.

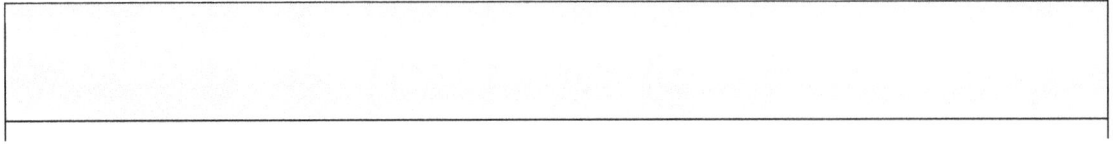

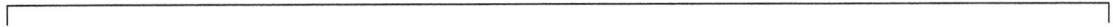

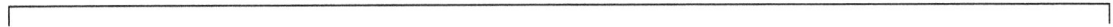

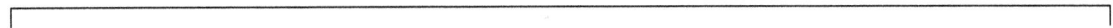

References

Aagaard, M (2003), *Workout,* Aagaard

Aagaard, M (2009), *Fitness og styrketræning,* Aagaard

ACE (2000), *Group Fitness Instructor Manual,* ACE

ACE (2004), *Group Strength Training,* ACE

Anderson, B (1980), *Stretching,* Clausen Bøger

Beier, T (1999(, *On Top of the Ball (video),* MTB

Botonietz, K, Strange, D 1998, Use of Swiss Balls in athletic training, *IAAF quarterly,* no.2

Boyle, M (2004), *Functional Conditioning for Sports,* Human Kinetics

Carriére, B (1998), *The Swiss Ball,* Springer

Chek, PW (2000), *Movement that matters,* CHEK Institute

Cibrario, M (1997), *Resistance exercises,* SPRI Products, Inc.

Cunningham, C (2002), Stability ball Training, Healthy Learning

Delavier, F (2001, *Strength Training Anatomy,* Human Kinetics

DIF (2005), *Muskeltraening,* DIF

Goldenberg, L, Twist, P (2007), *Strength Ball Training,* Human Kinetics

Gymnic, Active Dynamic Sitting, *Review of Sit'n'Gym findings*

Hodel, P, Balls and chairs in classrooms, *New Med*/Ledraplastic

Kempf, H-D, *Trainingsbuch Fitnessball,* Ro Ro Ro

Miller, G, *Extreme Training on the Ball (video),* Ground Control

Mitchell, C (2003), *Yoga on the Ball,* Healthy Arts Press

Morris, M 1998, Training on the Ball, *IDEA Personal Trainer,* nov-dec, p. 19-23

Rado, L (2001), *Yoga on the Ball (video),* Hugger mugger

Santana, JC (1999), *The Essence of Stability ball Training,* Optimum Performance

Sutherland, V 1999, Yoga on the Ball, *IDEA Source,* no. 4

Simonsen, O, Larsen, A S, Kaalund, S (1995), *All-Round Fitness,* Centrum

Glossary

Ab curl	Flexion of the spine, exercise.
Abduction	Away from the midline of the body.
Adduction	Towards the midline of the body.
Agonist	The primary working muscle of the movement.
Antagonist	The muscle with the opposite function of the agonist.
Anterior	Nearer the front.
Barbell	Bar for weight plates.
Bent-over	Leaning forward, forward flexion (rows, etc.).
Bilateral	With both arms or legs.
Circumduktion	Circular movement.
Closed-chain	Training with distal segment anchored.
Concentric	Muscle contraction, the muscle shortens.
Contraction	Muscle work, the muscle shortens or lengthens.
Continuus	Action carries on without stopping or interruption.
Coordination	Neuro-muscular function.
Core training	Working the muscles between the pelvic floor and the diaphragm.
Curl	Bend, flex.
Crunch	Ab curl with pelvis and torso curling up at the same time.
Decline	Lying at an angle with the head downwards.
Dorsal	Towards the back of the body, foot or hand.
Dumbbell	A small bar with weight plates.
Eccentric	Muscle contraction, the muscle lengthens.
Elevation	Lifting.
Eversion	Outward rotation, the sole of the foot outwards.
Extension	Straightening.
Flex	Bend. Contract muscle.
Flexion	Bending.
Flys	The arms in horizontal plane making an embracing movement.
Frontal plane	Plane from shoulder to shoulder, lateral movements.
Functional training	Any training that has a function for sports or every day living.
Horizontal plane	Plane transversing the body, also transversal plane.
Hyperextension	Extending further than neutral, normal, position.

Glossary

Incline	Lying at an angle with the head upwards.
Inversion	Inward rotation, the sole of the foot turns in.
Isometric	Muscle contraction without joint movement.
Lateral	To the side, away from the midline of the body.
Ligament	Strong tissue connecting bone to bone.
Lumbar	Concerning the lower part of the back/spine.
Lunge	Stepping forward or out, exercise.
Medial	Towards the midline of the body.
Open-chain	Training with distal segment moving freely (not anchored).
Overload	Increased load for continued progression.
Palmar	Towards the palm of the hand.
Partial	Smaller, limited range of motion.
Plantar	Towards the sole of the foot.
Plié	Squat with legs wide apart.
Prone	Lying face down.
Pronated	Hands or feet turned inwards/downwards.
Posterior	Placed behind or at the back.
Plyometrics	Explosive strength training, focus on the speed component.
Pronation	Hands of feet turned inward/downward.
Repetition	One complete move, concentric and eccentric phase
Rotation	Turning around an axis (left, right, medially, laterally).
Resistance band	Long flat piece of rubberband for resistance training.
Sagittal plane	From the back to the front, movementr forward/backward.
Sit-up	Abdominal curl with hip flexion (the torso comes up to the legs).
Spotter	A helper, who observes and assists during strength training.
Squat	Bending the legs, lowering the body. A classic functional exercise.
Supine	Lying face up.
Supination	Hands or feet turned outward/upward.
Synergist	Muscle working together with the agonist to perform the movement.
Set	A number of repetitions performed in sequence without a pause.
Tube	Long round (approx. 1,2 m) piece of rubbertube for resistance training.
Unilateral	With one arm or leg at a time.

About the Author

Marina Aagaard, *Master of Fitness and Exercise,* part-time associate professor at Aalborg University, Sports, and former head of the Fitness Department at the Coaching Academy of Denmark, 1995-2010, National Coach of Aerobic Gymnastics and consultant to the Danish Gymnastics Federation, 1995-2008.

Before that she served as a regional aerobics manager and health club manager for the Form and Figur health club chain. From 1991 she co-owned and managed the family health club, BodyTeria, Aarhus, as well as working as a consultant and lecturer at her fitness company aagaard.

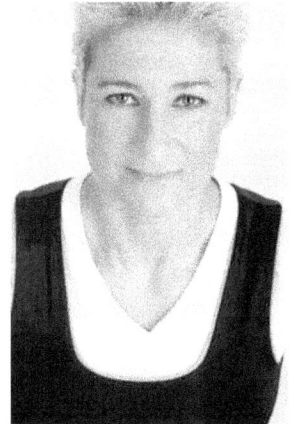

Marina is a certified Holistic Lifestyle Coach, CHEK Institute, as well as American Council on Exercise certified group exercise instructor and personal trainer (gold).

For seven years she was head of the Danish Reebok Instructor Club and became a Step and Slide Reebok Master Trainer. Together with Gin Miller, the inventor of steptraining, she starred in the 1993-1994 Eurosport Step Reebok series.

At the same time Marina created and hosted her own morning aerobic TV-series as well as choreographing numerous aerobic and dance shows and performances for national television.

Her interest in elite training led to choreographing, coaching and judging at aerobics and fitness competions. Marina served as an Aerobic Gymnastics judge, Juge Breveté, for the FIG, the International Gymnastics Federation, and judged at every European and World Championship from 1995-2004.

For more than 25 years she has been involved in strength training and conditioning of recreational exercisers as well as world class athletes.

Marina has published numerous articles on fitness and is the author of a series of fitness books and more than 100 compendia on resistance training and group exercise.

Marina enjoys strength training, group exercise, running, skiing and skating as well as music, dance, art, cars and travelling. She and her husband, Henrik, reside in the bay area of Kalø Vig, Jutland, Denmark.

Fitness Books

Resistance Training Exercises – Fitness and performance exercises

337 pages

The number one resource for resistance training exercises. It is all about exercises and variations. From simple isolations to advanced multi-exercisesfor one-on-one or group resistance training, for recreational or Olympic athletes.

With bodyweight, dumbbells, barbells, rubberbands,, tubes and bands. Also a great section on partner exercises. Comprehensive tables of more than 500 exercises, illustrated with over 1000 photos plus descriptions and notes.

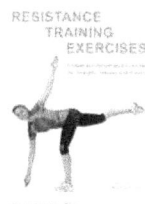

Stability ball Exercises – Fitness and performance exercisess

358 pages

The number one resource for stability ball exercises for everyone using the stability ball; coaches, trainers, instructors, physiotherapists, chiropractors and PE teachers.

For one-on-one fitness, group exercise and sports and physical exercise, for recreational exercisers to Olympic class athletes. The book contains comprehensive tables of more than 450 exercises, illustrated with more than 900 photos plus descriptions and notes.

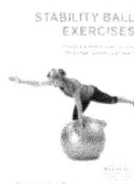

Aerobic – Functional Group Exercise in Theory and Practice, 6th Ed.

344 pages, Danish

A bestselling book on all aspects of aerobics and group exercise in general.

Based on research and practical experience within all modalities of international group exercise, this text is a must for anyone working with group exercise. An indispensable manual on: Music, sound, choreography, teaching methods and organization.

Including a complete guide to aerobic and dance aerobic steps.

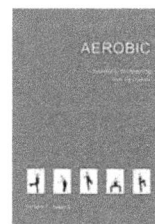

Step aerobics – four steps to optimal step training

264 pages, Danish

A popular textbook on everything you need to know about step training; the step, safety tips, correct stepping technique, various forms of step training. All about functional stepping – via intensity, impact and choreography.Including a comprehensive step guide, with more than 400 photos illustrating all basic steps and variations.

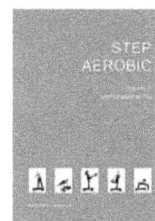

Workout – Group Resistance Training with Bodyweight or Equipment

235 pages, Danish

A popular textbook on resistance training, programmeming, exercises, sequencing and exercise technique. From isolation exercisesto complex, multi-exercises and functional training, for one-on-one and group resistance training, for beginning to advanced level. Designing workouts with bodyweight and equipment, including warm-up, balance work and core training. Including a comprehensive illustrated guide to exercises with bodyweight, barbells, dumbbells, tubes, bands, XerBars and UltraToners.

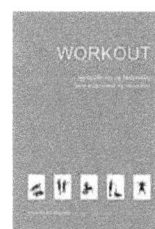

Spining, Biking & Cycling – Indoor Group Cycling in Theory and Practice

214 pages, Danish

An excellent handbook on one of the most popular forms of group exercise, group indoor cycling. For instructors and trainers. All about the indoor bike, setting up the bike, cycling equipment and riding technigue. Cardiovascular training and heart rate monitoring. In-depth descriptions of all parts of the group cycling class plus use of music and drills. Numerous ideas fordrills and teaching methods. Including 20 complete programmes.

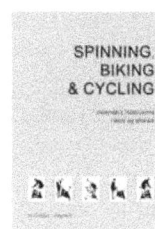

www.ingramcontent.com/pod-product-compliance
Lightning Source LLC
Chambersburg PA
CBHW080841270326
41927CB00013B/3058